Sleep Better and Less - Naturally: Cure Chronic Insomnia and Boost Body-Brain O2 Levels

Artour Rakhimov

Copyright

Disclaimer

TABLE OF CONTENTS

Copyright.. 2
Disclaimer 2
Introduction 5
1. MEDICAL EVIDENCE RELATED TO SLEEP AND EFFECTS OF HEAVY BREATHING 8
1.1 Sleep Heavy Breathing Effect: highest mortality rates...................... 8
1.2 Breathing in severely sick and critically ill people............................ 19
1.3 Other clinical and physiological facts... 26
1.4 The crucial role of the morning CP (Control Pause) in your health restoration 29
1.5 When the CP drops down to the lower health zone 32
1.6 You need to measure and record your morning CP and other CP numbers 33
1.7 How to analyze your morning CP drop.. 34
1.8 The morning CP miracle effect, or why morning CP matters 37
1.9 The morning CP test is a compromise.. 38
1.10 Your morning CP: the key factor of your quality of sleep 39
2. WHICH SLEEP FACTORS CAUSE HEALTH PROBLEMS 41
2.1 Sleeping too long 41
2.2 Wrong sleep positions.. 41
2.3 Mouth breathing 46
2.4 Electrical insulation from the Earth.. 51
2.5 The domino effect due to poor sleep... 53
2.6 Chest breathing 55
2.7 Too warm conditions 58
2.8 Soft beds 59
3. WHICH OTHER FACTORS MAKE SLEEP WORSE AND REDUCE MORNING CP? ... 60
3.1 Late supper.. 60
3.2 A lack of physical exercise... 60
3.3 Nutritional deficiencies.. 61
3.4 A lack of cortisol... 62
3.5 Acute exacerbations... 62
4. BLUEPRINT OF ACTIONS AND FIRST CRUCIAL STEPS...................................... 64
4.1 How to sleep less and better: the main goal...................................... 64
4.2 Best sleep positions.. 65
4.3 How to ensure nose breathing 69
4.4 How to ground yourself... 74
4.5 Eliminating the domino effect... 81
4.6 Chest breathing 85

4.7 Too warm conditions *86*
4.8 Soft beds *87*
4.9 Sleep restriction *87*
5. ADDITIONAL SLEEP FACTORS *95*
5.1 Earlier supper *95*
5.2 Reduced eating especially if you are overweight *95*
5.3 Physical exercise for shorter and better sleep *96*
5.4 Diet, nutrition and supplements *97*
5.5 Cold shower before sleep and during the day *98*
5.6 Walk in fresh air *99*
6. EXAMPLES OF SLEEP POSITIONS AND SWADDLING *100*
6.1 Horizontal sleep postures *100*
6.2 Sitting sleep positions *101*
6.3 Swaddling for people with very low morning CPs *108*
6.4 Using 2 or more belts for swaddling during sleep *110*
6.5 Degree of swaddling and morning CP *114*
6.6 Criteria and area for swaddling *114*
6.7 Type of belts for swaddling *116*
6.8 How to make a swaddling vest *120*
6.9 Best swaddling vest (a new method) *134*
6.10 Possible problems due to swaddling *139*
6.9 Three major factors that make swaddling easier to tolerate *141*
6.10 Crucial rules related to swaddling *142*
7. QUESTIONS AND ANSWERS ABOUT SLEEP, SYMPTOMS, AND BREATHING *144*
7.1 Sleep stages and duration of sleep *144*
7.2 Swaddling during sleep *149*
7.3 Overbreathing during sleep *150*
7.5 Sleep conditions *152*
7.6 Sleep positions *155*
7.7 Sleep and breathing in world class athletes *160*
Recommended reading *163*
Other books by Dr. Artour Rakhimov *164*

Introduction

Millions of people believe in a myth that the human body recovers or heals itself during sleep. This healing-sleep fantasy can be found in hundreds of books and internet articles on sleep.

Scientific evidence suggests the exact opposite scenario: for most people, the main damage to health is done during sleep. Every year millions of people have acute exacerbations of their conditions during sleep. Furthermore, numerous studies have shown that the highest mortality rates and highest chances of acute attacks are during early morning hours. This relates to asthma and COPD exacerbations, coronary spasms and cardiac arrest (or heart attacks), angina pectoris, strokes, cerebral ischemia, epilepsy seizures, worsened blood glucose control and increased inflammation. This book quotes over 15 clinical studies that discovered this effect. In fact, to my knowledge, each medical study that tried to find the worst time of the day with the most health problems and symptoms found the same result.

How can the body heal itself during sleep if severely sick people are most likely to die during early morning hours and even ordinary people feel the worst in the morning? Therefore, sleep is a confusing, myth-laden area which is misunderstood by ordinary people, medical doctors and most alternative health practitioners. Sleep makes health worse and is the key factor that promotes the advance of chronic diseases.

Clinical experience of hundreds of Buteyko breathing practitioners suggests a similar conclusion. Sleep makes health problems worse for ordinary people and people with diseases. After testing more than 250,000 people, over 180 Soviet and Russian doctors found that it is also common to have the lowest results for the simple DIY body oxygen test (see instructions below) during early morning hours or after waking up.

These Soviet and Russian medical professionals, who applied the Buteyko method on their patients, explained the causes of worsening

5

health problems during sleep and suggested simple specific techniques to deal with this challenge related to sleep. I am referring to Buteyko breathing doctors who applied the Buteyko breathing method on more than 250,000 people in the USSR and Russia.

According to these doctors, there are simple, down-to-Earth causes or factors that lead to poorer health during sleep. One of these destructive factors is mouth breathing. Patients need to prevent mouth breathing during sleep. This can be achieved with easy mouth-taping techniques or some other methods. It is also necessary to prevent supine sleep or sleeping on one's back. There are easy-to-implement methods to accomplish this goal. Grounding the human body to Earth (also called "Earthing") is an additional initial step to prevent heavy breathing and low body oxygenation during sleep.

In contrast with these basic and logical ideas, most official Western internet sources suggest supine sleep as the best sleeping position. This is in spite of the fact that all sleep-related studies (I am referring to 24 studies, which compared the effects of different sleeping positions on the health state and symptoms of people with various health problems) found that the supine position was the worst sleep posture.

Modern medicine and family physicians also ignore the effects of mouth breathing. You can visit your family physician or general practitioner and do a simple test. Show that you have mouth breathing, describe your poor health and ask him or her about solutions. Less than 1% of doctors would suggest that you start or try nose breathing. Doctors do not learn, in medical schools, even basic things related to sleep and management of diseases.

The next popular myth relates to thermoregulation during sleep. The common perception is that the human body requires warm and cozy conditions for better sleep. However, practical evidence again suggests the opposite observations. Overheating during sleep is a serious health hazard that promotes mouth breathing and supine sleep leading to heavy breathing and low body oxygenation. Soft beds encourage hours of immobility during sleep, restricted blood flow to certain body parts and gradually intensified respiration.

Apart from these lifestyle factors, Soviet and Russian Buteyko doctors, while working with severely sick and hospitalized patients, developed several other techniques that help a person to "survive" through the night and have much better day-time wellbeing and performance. This book considers and describes these how-to-sleep methods and explains various other effects related to sleep.

1. Medical evidence related to sleep and effects of heavy breathing

This Chapter provides results of clinical studies related to acute exacerbations and mortality during sleep, and effects of overbreathing on the body.

1.1 Sleep Heavy Breathing Effect: highest mortality rates

The Sleep Heavy Breathing Effect explains decades of medical research and clinical observations that highest mortality rates for asthma, angina pectoris, stroke, seizures, and many other conditions are during sleep and especially the early morning hours (4-7 am). Let us review this research.

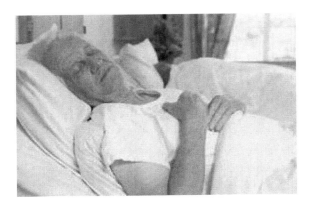

Asthma

American pediatricians from the Washington University School of Medicine in St. Louis in their publication noted,

"BACKGROUND: Symptoms from asthma are often prominent at night. In adults significant circadian variation has been shown with reduced peak expiratory flow rates and increased bronchial reactivity to methacholine in the early morning hours" (Porter et al, 1999).

A group of Brazilian medical scientists investigated, according to their title *Morning-to-evening variation in exercise-induced bronchospasm* (Vianna et al, 2002). Their objective was "to compare morning and evening EIB [exercise-induced bronchospasm] and minute ventilation during exercise (VE)" (Vianna et al, 2002). Baseline FEV1 was significantly lower during early morning hours, while minute ventilation higher."

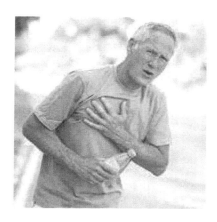

Over 30 years ago the Thorax published a study: *Physiological patterns in early morning asthma* (Hetzel, et al, 1977). The goal of the study was also to explain "the sudden nature of some asthma deaths as these often occur in the early morning" (Hetzel, et al, 1977).

COPD

Several other publications were devoted to effects of sleep on patients with COPD (chronic obstructive pulmonary disease). American scientists from the Yale Center for Sleep Medicine (Yale University School of Medicine, New Haven) wrote,

"Symptoms related to sleep disturbances are common in individuals with moderate to severe COPD, particularly in the elderly, which is commonly manifested as morning fatigue and early awakenings. One major cause of morbidity in this population is abnormalities in gas exchange and resultant hypoxemia as they can lead to elevated pulmonary pressures, dyspnea and in severe cases right ventricular overload and failure. Sleep has profound adverse effects on respiration and gas exchange in patients with COPD…" (Urbano & Mohsenin, 2006).

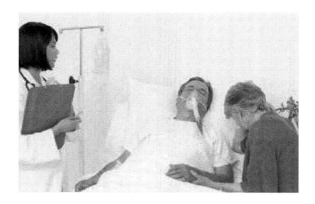

Moreover, Sheppard and colleagues in the publication from the Chest magazine noted, "Epidemiologic investigation has revealed that patients with pulmonary disease are at increased risk of dying during the early morning hours" (Sheppard et al, 1984). The load on the heart muscle during the episodes of hypoxemia during sleep, according to their conclusion, "can be transiently as great as during maximal exercise".

Coronary spasms and cardiac arrest

If patients with pulmonary conditions can die due to heart problems at night, what about heart patients themselves? "Coronary spasm occurs most often from midnight to early morning when the patient is at rest", (Yasue & Kugiyama, 1997) says the Japanese study *Coronary spasm: clinical features and pathogenesis* published in the Internal Medicine magazine. The main and only cause of these spasms is heavy breathing.

Intensive care professionals from the Department of Anesthesia and Intensive Care Medicine of the Hadassah Medical Centre in

Jerusalem, Israel, also decided to investigate, according to the study's title the following topic: *In-hospital cardiac arrest: is outcome related to the time of arrest?* They wrote,

"BACKGROUND: Whether outcome from in-hospital cardiopulmonary resuscitation (CPR) is poorer when it occurs during the night remains controversial. This study examined the relationship between CPR during the various hospital shifts and survival to discharge...CONCLUSIONS: Although unwitnessed arrest is more prevalent during night shift, resuscitation during this shift is associated with poorer outcomes independently of witnessed status" (Matot et al, 2006).

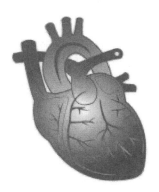

Trying to explain the cause of deaths, Turkish cardiologists from Ankara published a study with the title, *"Circadian variations of QTc dispersion: is it a clue to morning increase of sudden cardiac death?"* (The QTc interval is a measure of the time between the start of the Q wave and the end of the T wave in the heart's electrical cycle. A prolonged QT interval is a risk factor for ventricular tachyarrhythmias and sudden death.) They explained,

"BACKGROUND: Several studies related to cardiac events including sudden death have shown a peak incidence in the early morning hours. Our data suggest that QTcD has a circadian variation with an increase in the morning hours, especially in patients with coronary artery disease. This finding was thought to be an explanation for the role played by sympathetic nervous system in the occurrence of acute cardiac events and sudden death during these hours" (Batur et al, 1999).

A group of American cardiologists from the Georgetown University Medical Center in Washington, D.C. was also interested in the most likely time of death,

"The time of death was available in... 96 of the 139 patients who died suddenly. There was a circadian variation of all SCDs [sudden cardiac deaths] compared with other deaths with a distinct peak during the morning (p = 0.04)" (Behrens et al, 1997).

Angina pectoris

Swiss medical doctors explained in their abstract,

"Prinzmetal's angina is a variant of the classic exertion dependent angina pectoris. Typical is the appearance of the symptoms at rest during early morning hours. It is due to spasms in the coronary arteries. Various provocation tests may be used to trigger spasms, among others hyperventilation which leads to vasoconstriction of coronary arteries" (Jacob et al, 1994).

Stroke

Even healthy people have heavier breathing and lowered oxygenation of the brain during early morning hours, as Australian scientists from Latrobe University in Melbourne revealed. After testing healthy subjects, these scientists concluded,

"These data indicate that normal diurnal changes in the cerebrovascular response to $CO(2)$ influence the hypercapnic ventilatory response as well as the level of cerebral oxygenation during changes in arterial Pco(2); this may be a contributing factor for diurnal changes in breathing stability and the high incidence of stroke in the morning" (Cummings et al, 2007).

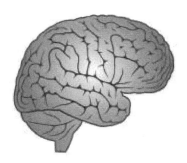

(Arterial Pco(2) means CO2 pressure in the arterial blood.)

These effects will cause symptoms of morning sickness fatigue or morning headache fatigue with possible adrenal fatigue and high morning cortisol.

Cerebral ischemia and stroke

It is not a surprise then that British researchers from the National Heart and Lung Institute (Imperial College, London) also noted,

"The reduction in hypercapnic cerebral vascular reactivity that occurs in the morning after sleep is associated with an increased risk of cerebral ischemia and stroke" (Meadows et al, 2005).

Similarly, Californian neurologists wrote,

"This reduced morning response to hypercapnia suggests diminished vasodilator reserve during this period, and may be related to the increased stroke risk during the morning hours" (Ameriso et al, 1994).

Diabetes

Patients with diabetes also suffer from lower oxygenation in tissues during nights:

"Circadian rhythms of tissue oxygen balance and blood rheological properties were investigated in 40 patients with insulin dependent diabetes mellitus... Preserved blood hyperviscosity and increasing tissue hypoxia at night indicated stable disturbance of hemorheological properties and tissue oxygen balance" (Galenok et al, 1988).

Seizures

Japanese doctors from the Department of Pathology for the Handicapped in Ehime University warn that those who care about people with epilepsy should know about higher chances of seizures during nights:

"...S-w paroxysms combined with clinical symptoms and continuing for more than four seconds were fewer during the afternoon than the morning and, moreover, during sleep. ...Therefore, the observation of typical absence seizures during the morning should be regarded as important" (Nagao et al, 1990).

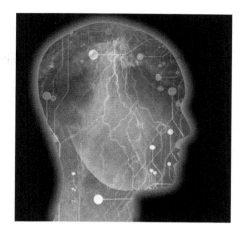

Since heavy breathing reduces blood supply and oxygenation of the brain, while also making nerve cells over-excited, it is sensible that epileptics are most likely to experience seizures during sleep (early morning hours).

Inflammatory conditions

A marker of inflammation, C-reactive protein, was measured during different parts of the day in obese patients (Punjabi & Beamer, 2007). The conclusion of these medical scientists from the Johns Hopkins University in Baltimore was in the title of the study, *C-reactive protein is associated with sleep disordered breathing independent of adiposity*. Hence, it is not just obesity, but disordered breathing at night that can lead to inflammation:

"...the results of this study suggest that mechanisms other than adiposity per se could contribute to the inflammatory state seen in adults with SDB [sleep disordered breathing]" (Punjabi & Beamer, 2007).

Inflammation in amnesic patients

Since inflammation can get worse during nights in many patients, is it possible that cortisol production (cortisol is one of the key hormones to fight inflammation) also decreases at nights? German researchers suggested,

"Some studies found patterns of enhanced or blunted waking cortisol responses observed under chronic stress, burnout, or post traumatic stress disorder... The morning cortisol increase typically observed in healthy subjects and also observed in the control group was absent in the amnesic patients... Further studies are needed to understand the neurological or psychological mechanisms leading to a missing morning cortisol response in amnesic patients" (Wolf et al, 2005).

Morning sickness

"Approximately two-thirds of women experience nausea or vomiting during the first trimester of pregnancy. These symptoms are commonly known as morning sickness" (Flaxman & Sherman, 2000).

It is known that pregnancy in modern women means even more chronic hyperventilation. Many of these women have even heavier breathing during sleep in comparison with their usual daily chronic hyperventilation. Hence, they often experience adrenal fatigue and high morning cortisol and morning headache fatigue.

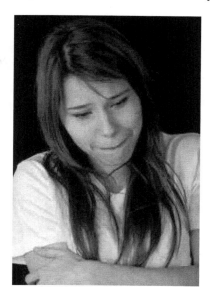

Conclusions

Most diseases appear and progress during early morning hours. Severely sick people are most likely to die during the same time of the day (about 4-7 am). The real health of the person can be only as good as their morning CP ("Control Pause" or the body oxygen test described below) measured immediately after waking up.

References

Ameriso SF, Mohler JG, Suarez M, Fisher M, Morning reduction of cerebral vasomotor reactivity, Neurology 1994 Oct; 44(10): 1907-1909.

Batur MK, Aksöyek S, Oto A, Yildirir A, Ozer N, Atalar E, Aytemir K, Kabakci G, Ovünç K, Ozmen F, Kes S, Circadian variations of QTc dispersion: is it a clue to morning increase of sudden cardiac death? Clin Cardiol. 1999 Feb; 22(2): 103-106.

Behrens S, Ney G, Fisher SG, Fletcher RD, Franz MR, Singh SN, Effects of amiodarone on the circadian pattern of sudden cardiac death, Am J Cardiol. 1997 Jul 1; 80(1): 45-48.

Dr. Artour Rakhimov

Cummings KJ, Swart M, Ainslie PN, Morning attenuation in cerebrovascular CO2 reactivity in healthy humans is associated with a lowered cerebral oxygenation and an augmented ventilatory response to CO2, J Appl Physiol. 2007 May; 102(5): 1891-1898. Flaxman SM, Sherman PW, Morning sickness: a mechanism for protecting mother and embryo, Q Rev Biol. 2000 Jun; 75(2): 113-148.

Galenok VA, Krivosheeva IA, Dikker VE, Krivosheev AB, Desynchronization of circadian rhythms of the oxygen balance in the tissues and rheological properties of the blood in type I diabetes mellitus [Article in Russian].

Hetzel MR, Clark TJ, Houston K, Physiological patterns in early morning asthma, Thorax 1977 Aug; 32(4): 418-423.

Jakob M, Hess OM, Mayer I, Hu Z, Krayenbühl HP, Prinzmetal's variant angina: a case report [Article in German], Schweiz Rundsch Med Prax. 1994 May 10; 83(19): 579-582.

Matot I, Shleifer A, Hersch M, Lotan C, Weiniger CF, Dror Y, Einav S, In-hospital cardiac arrest: is outcome related to the time of arrest? Resuscitation 2006 Oct; 71(1): 56-64.

Meadows GE, Kotajima F, Vazir A, Kostikas K, Simonds AK, Morrell MJ, Corfield DR, Overnight changes in the cerebral vascular response to isocapnic hypoxia and hypercapnia in healthy humans: protection against stroke, Stroke 2005 Nov; 36(11): 2367-2372.

Nagao H, Morimoto T, Takahashi M, Habara S, Nagai H, Matsuda H, The circadian rhythm of typical absence seizures--the frequency and duration of paroxysmal discharges, Neuropediatrics 1990 May; 21(2): 79-82.

Porter FL, White D, Attaway N, Miller JP, Strunk RC, Absence of diurnal variability of airway reactivity and hypoxic ventilatory drive in adolescents with stable asthma, J Allergy Clin Immunol. 1999 May; 103(5 Pt 1): 804-809.

18

Punjabi NM, Beamer BA, C-reactive protein is associated with sleep disordered breathing independent of adiposity, Sleep 2007 Jan 1; 30(1): 29-34.

Shepard JW Jr, Schweitzer PK, Keller CA, Chun DS, Dolan GF, Myocardial stress, Exercise versus sleep in patients with COPD, Chest 1984 Sep; 86(3): 366-374.

Urbano F, Mohsenin V, Chronic obstructive pulmonary disease and sleep: the interaction, Panminerva Med 2006 Dec; 48(4): 223-230.

Vianna EO, Boaventura LC, Terra-Filho J, Nakama GY, Martinez JA, Martin RJ, Morning-to-evening variation in exercise-induced bronchospasm, J Allergy Clin Immunol. 2002 Aug; 110(2): 236-240.

Wolf OT, Fujiwara E, Luwinski G, Kirschbaum C, Markowitsch HJ, No morning cortisol response in patients with severe global amnesia, Psychoneuroendocrinology 2005 Jan; 30(1): 101-105.

Yasue H, Kugiyama K, Coronary spasm: clinical features and pathogenesis, Intern Med. 1997 Nov; 36(11): 760-765.

1.2 Breathing in severely sick and critically ill people

"...Death consists of the passing out of the air. It is, therefore, necessary to restrain the breath."
Hatha Yoga Pradipika, Ancient Sanskrit text, 15th century.

It is a normal clinical finding that with approaching death, breathing becomes faster and deeper, while oxygen levels in the brain, heart and other vital organs decrease. Separate web pages of NormalBreathing.com provide medical references that confirm very high respiratory rates (fast and labored breathing, up to 30-50 breaths per minute at rest) in terminal cancer, last stages of HIV-AIDS, cystic fibrosis, and other conditions. (By the way, in the 1950's, observations of breathing patterns in dying hospitalized patients led Dr. Buteyko to the discovery of the mystery of death and creation of the Buteyko breathing method.)

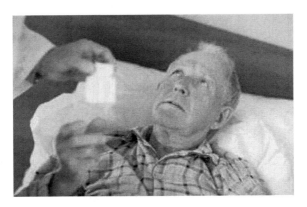

Many studies commented about and measured effects of heavy breathing on health states of different groups of patients.

For example, all 29 patients with severe liver damage (in most cases due to deadly metastatic cancer or cirrhosis of liver) had low arterial carbon dioxide, while for 25 patients "*it was also clinically evident that respiratory exchange was increased markedly*" (p.762, Wanamee et al, 1956). Thus, hyperventilation or heavy breathing was visually observed by the authors of the publication, *Respiratory alkalosis in hepatic coma*. They also found that very heavy, labored breathing led to severe electrolyte abnormalities. These abnormalities included decreased sodium ions and increased chloride ions in the blood. Abnormally high lactic and pyruvic acid concentrations were other frequent effects.

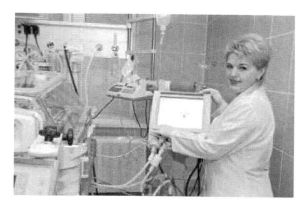

Blood gases and respiratory patterns provided accurate information for survival prognosis in acute cerebrovascular accidents. When these parameters were normal, patients survived. Out of 11 hyperventilating patients with less than 35 mm Hg arterial CO_2, only one survived (Rout et al, 1971).

The same conclusion (regarding arterial CO_2 and survival prognosis) was made for head injuries (Huang et al, 1963; Vapalanti & Trouph, 1971).

Summarizing the results of these works and their connection with brain dysfunction, Dr. Plum wrote,

"The combination of hyperpnoea [increased breathing] with an elevated pH, and a subnormal or moderately low oxygen tension occurs in many serious illnesses that entirely spare the brain. These include the alveolar-capillary block of diffuse pulmonary carcinomatosis; heart failure; advanced cirrhosis, with or without hepatic coma; acute pulmonary infarction; and many others, including the cryptic pulmonary congestion that accompanies most serious disease in the obtunded and elderly" (Plum, 1972).

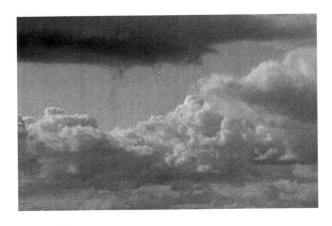

Interestingly, all above-mentioned effects (low carbon dioxide concentration, elevated pH, and hypoxia or low O2 pressure in cells) quoted by Dr. Plum are caused by heavy breathing.

As a result, one can conclude that labored breathing is a normal feature of these severe diseases.

When suffering various serious health problems (heart disease, diabetes, cancer, AIDS, etc.) the patient's life is usually threatened, not by the main health problem, but by complications and infections, such as in the case of bacteremic shock. Analyzing a group of patients initially diagnosed with arteriosclerotic heart disease, cerebrovascular insufficiency, diabetes, arthritis, several forms of cancer, fatty liver, and alcoholism, one study showed that complications due to pathogenic microorganisms in the blood caused 46 deaths in 50 patients (Winslow et al., 1973). Pneumonia and urinary tract infections were the foci of pathogenic microorganisms. Now we may ask the following: what was observed with their breathing, when not only a part of the organism, but even the blood was polluted with pathogens? All 50 patients, according to a table accompanying this article, had very disturbed blood gases corresponding to very labored breathing.

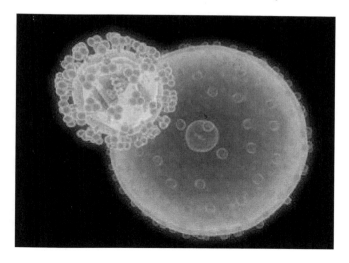

Dr. Simmons and his colleagues wrote an article, "Hyperventilation and respiratory alkalosis as signs of gram-negative bacteremia" (bacteremia being the presence of bacteria in the blood). This excerpt is from the beginning of their abstract:

"Visible hyperventilation was observed clinically in patients with Gram-negative bacteremia. Eleven patients with Gram-negative infections and either proved or probable bacteremias were therefore studied to see if hyperventilation might be a common response to such bacteremia. In every case there was laboratory evidence of hyperventilation, and in 8 cases the hyperventilation was visible to the observer. Since only patients were studied who had no other cause for increased ventilation, this appears to be a primary response to the bacteremia..." (abstract, Simmons et al, 1960).

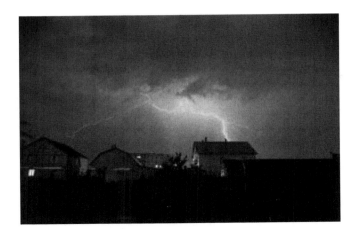

Another group of US medical professionals found that the degree of heavy breathing has a strong correlation with overall mortality (Mazarra et al, 1974). Heavier breathing indicated smaller chances of survival. Here is what they wrote in their scientific abstract:

"Through a retrospective review of the randomly selected hospital records of 114 patients, we defined four groups based upon arterial carbon dioxide tension ($PaCO_2$) and mode of ventilation. Group I, with a $PaCO_2$ of 15 mm Hg or less, consisted of 25 patients with an over-all mortality of 88 per cent. Group II, with a $PaCO_2$ of 20 to 25 mm Hg, consisted of 35 patients with a mortality of 77 per cent. Group III, with a $PaCO_2$ of 25 to 30 mm Hg, consisted of 33 patients with a mortality of 73 per cent, and Group IV, with a $PaCO_2$ of 35 to 45 mm Hg, consisted of 21 patients with a mortality of 29 per cent ($p<0.001$). Shock and sepsis were most common in group I patients" (abstract, Mazarra et al, 1974).

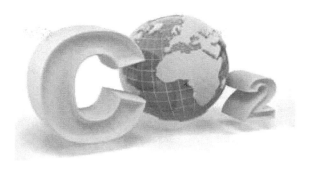

This article indicated that the most common diseases to occur in all 4 groups of people were cerebrovascular disease, hepatic coma, bronchopneumonia, and arteriosclerotic heart disease.

A review of these professional studies indicates that critically ill patients usually have very low carbon dioxide levels due to visible hyperventilation. Labored breathing (the heavy breathing pattern) of such patients corresponds to minute ventilation of 20-25 liters of air per minute or more, while the norm for breathing at rest is only 6 l/min.

The analysis of Western medical literature suggests that many critically ill patients die in conditions of heavy and deep breathing. Up to 90% of deaths in the severely sick take place when breathing becomes progressively heavier and deeper, while the CP gradually approaches zero.

Conclusions

Over 90% of people die in conditions of very heavy breathing causing critically low levels of CO2 in the blood and other body cells. Also, most exacerbations take place during early morning hours. Since early morning hours are the most likely time of these acute attacks and deaths, heavy breathing is one of the key risk factors that contributes to health misery during sleep. In fact, we are going to prove that overbreathing is the central factor that causes low body oxygenation and numerous other negative effects leading to worsened health in sick people and even relatively healthy individuals.

References

Huang CT, Cook AW, Lyons HA, Severe cranio cerebral trauma and respiratory abnormalities, Arch Neurol 1963, 9: p. 545-554.

Mazarra JT, Ayres SM, Grace WJ, Extreme hypocapnia in the critically ill patient, Amer J Med Apr 1974, 56: p. 450-456.

Plum F, Hyperpnea, hyperventilation and brain dysfunction, Annals of Intern Med 1972, 76: p. 328.

Rout MW, Lane DJ, Wolliner L, Prognosis in acute cerebrovascular accidents in relation to respiratory pattern and blood gas tension, Br Med J 1971, 3: p. 7-9.

Simmons DH, Nicoloff J, Guze LB, Hyperventilation and respiratory alkalosis as signs of gram-negative bacteremia, J Amer Med Assoc 1960, 174: p. 2196-2199.

Vapalanti M & Troup H, Prognosis for patients with severe brain injuries, Br Med J 1971, 3: p. 404-407.

Wanamee P, Poppel JW, Glicksman AS, Randall HT, Roberts KE, Respiratory alkalosis in hepatic coma, Arch Intern Med 1956, 97: p. 762-767.

1.3 Other clinical and physiological facts

There are many other physiological facts and ideas that are important to learn in order to improve your health. Let me review some of these facts and ideas.

1. The physiological norm for breathing at rest (for a 70-kg man) corresponds to:

- 6 l/min for minute ventilation
- 12 breaths/min for breathing frequency
- 500 ml for tidal volume (amount of air for one breath)
- 98% oxygen saturation for the arterial blood
- 40 mm Hg (or 5.3%) CO_2 partial pressure in the arterial blood and alveoli
- 40 seconds for the BHT (breath holding time) test done after usual exhalation and without any stress during and after the test (i.e., without pushing yourself for better numbers).

2. The special breath holding time test, which is called the CP (control pause), is the most accurate DIY test to measure breathing and body oxygenation. You need to find web pages or videos that explain how to do this CP test, and practice this test every morning.

3. Ordinary modern people breathe about 12 l/min at rest (numerous published studies) or about 2 times more than the norm established about 100 years ago. People do not notice when they breathe up to 2-3 times more than the medical norm.

4. Mildly sick people breathe about 12-18 l/min or about 2-3 times more than the norm (numerous published medical studies), while their body oxygenation is below the norm, and the CP is less than 20 s.

5. Severely sick, critically ill, and hospitalized patients have even heavier breathing and even less oxygen in their bodies (less than 10 s for the CP).

6. When we breathe more than the norm (hyperventilation or overbreathing), we do not increase oxygenation of the arterial blood (see above). The main effect of hyperventilation is excessive removal of CO_2 from the lungs, blood and cells. This causes:
- constriction of arteries and arterioles (CO_2 is a powerful vasodilator)
- the suppressed Bohr effect (reduced release of oxygen by red blood cells in tissues due to less CO_2).
As a result, all vital organs (including, the brain, heart, kidneys,

liver, pancreas, large and small intestines, stomach, spleen, etc.) get less blood and oxygen supply.

7. Hence, the more one breathes at rest the less oxygen he or she gets. The details of this relationship can be found in the Buteyko Table of Health Zones. This Table links major physiological parameters, such as CO_2 levels in the lungs, the CP result, breathing frequency, and heart rate.

8. The "goodness of deep breathing" propaganda, as presented by TV, newspapers, radio, and other mass media, when it is applied to unconscious or basal breathing, is falsehood based on ignorance and lack of education in basics of physiology and respiration. Most modern yoga teachers, yoga websites, sports coaches and fitness instructors, as well as some official medical sources, also promote the same myth.

9. Basal or unconscious breathing at rest becomes heavier (faster and deeper) and body oxygenation less due to:
- Lack of physical exercise
- Mouth breathing (including during sleep and physical exercise, unless you are super fit)
- Sleeping on one's back and too much sleep
- Psychological stress, anger, revenge, greed, envy, jealousy, laziness, and strong emotions
- Overeating (especially of animal proteins)
- Overheating
- Lack of essential nutrients; junk foods
- Toxins and pollution (in water, food and air, due to radiation, infections, and medical drugs); allergens; dusty environment
- Poor posture (slouching is present in over 90% of modern people)
- Talkativeness and deep breathing exercises (except very slow ones, e.g., with 1-2 breaths/min so as to get more CO_2)
- Sighing, coughing, sneezing and yawning with large air movements or open mouth
- Excesses and addictions (smoking, street drugs, gambling, too much alcohol, caffeine, sunbathing, sex, etc.)

10. Basal or unconscious breathing at rest becomes easier (lighter and slower) and body oxygenation higher due to:
- Physical exercise with strictly nasal breathing (in and out) due to increased CO_2 and nitric oxide concentrations
- Forgiveness and silent prayer; relaxation and meditation exercises; peace-making, good will, cooperation, self-discipline, perseverance, commitment, and responsibility
- Good posture (straight spine 24/7)
- More time outdoors (especially for the aged)
- Eating only when really hungry, and stopping in time
- Going to bed for sleep, only when really sleepy, and getting out of bed after waking up in the morning; sleeping on hard beds
- Raw vegetarian diet (only if very well chewed)
- Moderation in pleasures, cold shower (with certain rules), barefoot walking, massage
- Some breathing exercises (the Buteyko method, Frolov breathing device, Breathslim, DIY breathing device, Strelnikova paradoxical breathing gymnastic, correctly done pranayama, and so forth)

These are only some of the negative and positive lifestyle factors. There are nearly a hundred more. In this book, we are going to focus on those factors that relate to sleep.

For hundreds of medical studies that confirm the above physiological laws and facts, visit NormalBreathing.com.

1.4 The crucial role of the morning CP (Control Pause) in your health restoration

I assume that you have already measured your body O2 levels using the CP (Control Pause) test many times, including your morning CP. If not, start doing it up to 10 or more times per day. The instructions for the CP test are simple. They can be found on YouTube and the internet: http://www.normalbreathing.com/index-measure-CP.php.

Morning CP instructions are relatively simple:
When you open your eyes in the morning or just before you get out of bed, make your usual exhalation, pinch the nose, and do the CP

test (but only until the very first or very initial signs of stress) while still in bed. Be prepared that the morning CP result is less, sometimes much less, than your usual evening CP numbers.

Probably you are wondering which CP number is most important for breathing retraining. This question is very important since the answer and the corresponding attitude shape the strategy and chosen activities.

Some Buteyko breathing method practitioners greatly emphasize the importance of many breathing sessions and an ability to achieve very large CP numbers during the day. These are great things. This can be called a CP-aggressive approach. However, it is even more important to maintain the same level of health during and after sleep. Why is it so important?

During the night we cannot directly control our breathing. For most people, as was discussed before, breathing is heaviest between about 3 and 7 am. The CP is lowest during these early morning hours. Meanwhile, the main damage to the body, with resetting of the breathing centre, corresponds to the minimum daily CP. Many positive changes could be eliminated. The rate of progress is reduced. The student has to start over almost from the beginning. This is the reason why I started this book with clinical studies related to Sleep Heavy Breathing Effect or morning hyperventilation. Conclusions: **severely sick people are most likely to have acute exacerbations or even die during early morning hours (4-7 am), when our breathing is heaviest and body oxygenation lowest. This fact was found for heart disease, stroke, COPD, asthma, epilepsy and many other conditions.**

Imagine, for example, what happens when your morning CP is very low.

If you have asthma and hyperventilate during early morning hours (as most asthmatics do), oxygenation of the body is critically low, airways become constricted and irritated, and more inflammation is produced. Your body will try to repair inflammation in airways during the day, when the CP is higher. But if you hyperventilate every morning, or even every other morning, healing of airways will never take place. There is simply not enough time to heal since the damage is systematically done.

It is the same as scratching a wound every day until it bleeds and then hoping that it will go away one day. Surely, an asthmatic cannot expect a real health breakthrough if he suffers from morning hyperventilation manifested in his or her low morning CP and increased airway inflammation.

If you have congenital heart disease or other abnormalities in the heart muscle, the situation is the same. You will produce considerable damage to your heart tissue once your CP becomes less than 10 seconds. Later you may have the best breathing exercises, perfect diet, most wonderful supplements, and many other great things, but if you hyperventilate every morning, there is no health system that can help you to be healthier in the long run.

If you have cancer and your morning CP is lower than your usual CP numbers, then your tumor will grow and even metastasize during the early morning hours. Later, you can have the best diets, use the greatest supplements, get great physical exercise, and do many other useful things which can reduce your tumor, but, if your tumor grows by about 2 mm during 2-3 hours of morning hyperventilation and then shrinks by 1 mm during the remaining part of the day, what would be the total effect in 1-2 months?

Whatever health problem or concern you have, it is going to get worse and progress during the periods of lowest body oxygenation. This relates to malignant and benign tumors, any inflamed tissues or body parts (in your airways, digestive system, liver, kidneys, prostate, and so forth), and many other abnormalities, such as fluid in lungs, ear, knee or brain; granulomas in the lungs or stomach; lymphomas of the stomach, head, neck, brain or skin; glaucoma and cataracts and so forth.

The body has reserves to eliminate these abnormalities but only in conditions of normal or nearly normal:
- CO2 and O2 levels in cells
- blood flow or perfusion of tissues and organs.

Therefore, hyperventilation "feeds" all body abnormalities, making them worse. Even if you do not suffer from any detected or known chronic disease, but still have low morning CP (below 20 seconds), you still generate free radicals and cause damage to body cells due to tissue hypoxia and other effects of hyperventilation. Just 20-30 minutes of overbreathing with low CO2 in the lungs is enough to cause more damage.

1.5 When the CP drops down to the lower health zone

Furthermore, the negative effect related to the CP drop during sleep is present at higher CPs as well.

Assume that someone has problems with gastritis (inflammation of the stomach) or prostatitis (inflammation of the prostate gland). If this person gets about 35-40 s for the daily CPs, but his morning CPs are only about 25 seconds, he will produce enough damage due to this CP drop to make his inflammation permanent. In order to eliminate inflammation, this person needs to get 30+ seconds in the morning and maintain it for about 2-3 weeks.

Lowered morning CP causes damage to the body even when one's morning CP is up to 35-37 seconds. This situation takes place in breathing students who can get up to 50-60 seconds during the day due to breathing exercises and physical activity. However, these students often experience negative health changes that take place every morning due to the transition from a higher CP zone (more than 40 seconds), to a lower CP zone (less than 40 s).

Some Russian and Soviet Buteyko practitioners claim that this effect is present even at much higher CP levels (or up to 70-90 seconds), but in a much smaller degree. In other words, morning CP drop causes damage to healthier people, but to a smaller extent. Although there is less damage, a morning CP drop prevents these students from getting higher CP numbers.

For our purposes, since my goal is to guide you up to a 60 s morning CP, we are going to assume that there are 4 major thresholds or transitions between neighboring health zones in the Buteyko Table of Health Zones:

The morning CP drops below:	Effects of this morning CP drop:
10 seconds	People start to fight with death due to heart attacks, strokes, seizures, asthma and COPD exacerbations, etc.
20 seconds	Appearance of health symptoms that can range from coughing and blocked nose to chest pain and constipation
30 seconds	Growth or advance of malignant tumors, inflammation and other major tissue abnormalities
40 seconds	Growth of minor tissue abnormalities that consume resources of the body and worsen one's health keeping the CP below 40 s.

1.6 You need to measure and record your morning CP and other CP numbers

To find out the degree of this problem, every night, just before going to sleep, you should measure, if there are no contra-indications, the evening CP. It will tell about the progress you achieved during that particular day. The next step is to measure your morning CP and compare the result with your evening numbers.

After several days of measurements, there are many CP numbers in your daily log:
- the initial CPs before the breathing sessions
- the final CPs after the breathing sessions
- your morning CPs.

If you do a breathing session close to retiring to bed, then you can compare these numbers related to the breathing sessions with the morning CP numbers. If you do not have any results related to CP numbers after your last large meal or before sleep (usually supper), then you can also measure your CP before going to sleep. It can be done 5, 10 or 30 minutes before going to sleep.

1.7 How to analyze your morning CP drop

Your next goal is to analyze your numbers and find out the emerging pattern related to your personal circadian CP changes. Is the morning CP much smaller than the previous evening CP? By how much?

Some people have relatively short sleep (e.g., about 6 hours) even when their CPs are about 10 s or less. Usually these people do not have problems with lowered morning CP. Their morning CPs are nearly the same as their evening CP values. However, this is true only for a small number of people (about 10-20 %).

Practice shows that over 50% of modern people and most breathing students have a large CP drop: at least 30% or more during nighttime sleep. For example, the relative drop from 20 seconds to 14 seconds is exactly 30%. (To get 30%, you need to divide 14 by 20 and multiply the result by 100%. This gives you 70%. Therefore, the morning CP is only 70% of the evening CP. Hence, the CP drop is 30% in relative values and 6 seconds on absolute values.) For some of these people, the drop is even more drastic. Only a small proportion of people (less than 10-20%) have almost no difference (e.g., 1-2 s) between their evening and morning CP values.

Let me provide here a daily log and the way to analyze the morning CP drop. This is a snapshot of the daily log of one of my breathing students.

Date	MCP	Time (hour)	Init. pulse	Init. CP	Breath cycle and session time	Final pulse	Final CP
16 March		20:15	65	13	3s/18s, 20m	65	15
17 March	12	5:30	65	13	3s/18s, 20m	60	15
		19:30	75	10	3s/15s, 20m	70	16
18 March	10	6:45	66	12	3s/18s, 20m	66	14
		21:15				56	20
19 March	11	8:00		12	3s/19s, 20m	70	13
		17:30	76	11	3s/18s, 20m	61	16
20 March	12	8:30	65	12	3s/19s, 20m	55	13
		15:00	65	12	3s/19s, 20m	55	15
		20:00				51	15
21 March	13	7:30	55	13	3s/21s/20m	51	18
		21:00	54	17	3s/22s/20m	53	20
22 March	14	6:00	54	14	3s/22s/20m	49	15
		21:00	57	17	3s/23s/20m	54	20
23 March	14	7:00	54	15	3s/23s/20m	49	17
		19:30	57	17	3s/23s/20m	47	20
24 March	15	7:00	59	15	3s/23s/20m	51	17
		21:00	60	17	3s/24s/20m	50	19
25 March	16	8:00	60	15	3s/23s/20m	55	20
		21:00	56	17	3s/23s/20m	53	18
26 March	16	6:00	57	15	3s/24s/20m	54	22
		21:00	60	17	3s/24s/20m	51	20

For the sake of space (some reading devices cannot display large tables on one page), this daily log has the last 2 columns missing. They are about physical exercise and symptoms-medication-auxiliary activities. His breathing exercises were done with the Frolov breathing device.

A test for you: As a simple test, can you tell if this person has a serious problem with the morning CP drop? What are his typical CP drop numbers and relative CP drop?

The answer is relatively easy. You need to compare evening with next morning CP numbers. These numbers are circled on the next graph.

Date	MCP	Time (hour)	Init. pulse	Init. CP	Breath cycle and session time	Final pulse	Final CP
16 March		20:15	65	13	3s/18s, 20m	65	15
17 March	12	5:30	65	13	3s/18s, 20m	60	15
		19:30	75	10	3s/15s, 20m	70	16
18 March	10	6:45	66	12	3s/18s, 20m	66	14
		21:15				56	20
19 March	11	8:00		12	3s/19s, 20m	70	13
		17:30	76	11	3s/18s, 20m	61	16
20 March	12	8:30	65	12	3s/19s, 20m	55	13
		15:00	65	12	3s/19s, 20m	55	15
		20:00				51	15
21 March	13	7:30	55	13	3s/21s/20m	51	18
		21:00	54	17	3s/22s/20m	53	20
22 March	14	6:00	54	14	3s/22s/20m	49	15
		21:00	57	17	3s/23s/20m	54	20
23 March	14	7:00	54	15	3s/23s/20m	49	17
		19:30	57	17	3s/23s/20m	47	20
24 March	15	7:00	59	15	3s/23s/20m	51	17
		21:00	60	17	3s/24s/20m	50	19
25 March	16	8:00	60	15	3s/23s/20m	55	20
		21:00	56	17	3s/23s/20m	53	18
26 March	16	6:00	57	15	3s/24s/20m	54	22
		21:00	60	17	3s/24s/20m	51	20

We can see that on March 17, the CP dropped from 15 to 12 seconds, then, on the next day, from 16 to 10 seconds, from 20 to 11, from 16 to 12, from 15 to 13, from 20 to 14, again from 20 to 14, from 20 to 15, from 19 to 16, and, finally, from 18 to 16 seconds on March 26.

We can also glance at the right side and notice that the average evening CP is about 18 seconds, while the morning CP (on the left side of the log) is about 13-14 seconds. The morning CP drop is about 4.5 seconds or about 25% for the relative CP decrease. This is not so bad since many people have worse relative results.

We can also see that his overall CP progress is really good. His CP increased by about 5 seconds after practicing for slightly more than a week. He made this improvement with only 40 min per day for breathing exercises. Such CP progress is common in younger people who do more physical exercise (e.g., up to 1.5-2 hours per day), but rare in elderly people. This daily log is for a man who is 40+ years old.

If you have a larger drop in your morning CP (in comparison with the evening CP), this is not bad news at all. Why is this so? This is because this book provides you with exact details and instructions on how to increase your morning CP.

1.8 The morning CP miracle effect, or why morning CP matters

Let me return to the example provided above. What else can we see from his daily log?

We can notice that nearly all CP progress (due to breathing exercises) is eliminated or destroyed overnight, due to negative effects related to sleep. During the first several days for this log, the student increases his CP, due to breathing exercises, from about 12 to 16 seconds, but then his next morning CP decreases almost completely back to about 12 seconds.

What would happen if this person can cut this overnight CP decrease by half? He would get about 2 seconds more for his next morning CP, or about 14 seconds instead of 12. Note that these 2 seconds are not about his overall weekly CP increase. He would get this morning CP increase in 1 day. What progress can be expected in one week? In a week's time, he can expect over 10 seconds increase in his morning CP. This is a very large increase that is present in fewer than 3-5% of breathing students.

We can also imagine that this person does not have any overnight CP losses. Assume that he wakes up with the same morning CP number that he had for the previous evening CP. In this case, he will make astonishing overall CP progress: over 20 seconds in a week. This effect, when overnight CP drop is absent or very small, can be called "**the morning CP miracle**". In reality, due to "resistance" from the body (or due to the effects of body pollution, pathogens, inflamed tissues, poor digestive flora, and so on), the progress in sick and severely ill people can be significantly slower. However, whatever the health state of the person, the effects of the morning CP miracle are profound.

The goal of this discussion is to demonstrate that, for most people, the overnight CP drop plays the most crucial negative role in reduced overall CP growth and in reduced improvements in health. In other words, the average student spends a lot of time and energy on breathing exercises, physical activity and other beneficial activities, in order to increase his or her CP, but then the sleep comes, nearly all progress disappears or is erased.

Would the morning CP, after weeks of practice, improve, if breathing exercises and common sense activities are practiced? The experience of Buteyko practitioners shows that usually the person is still going to progress. However, it is obvious that an overnight CP drop is the greatest single factor impeding general CP progress and health restoration. It would make sense, therefore, to address the problem directly.

There is one more factor that actually makes the overnight CP drop even worse than our calculations.

1.9 The morning CP test is a compromise

As you should know, we measure the morning CP while still lying in the bed or in the horizontal position, while other CP numbers are measured while sitting. It is known that metabolism for the horizontal position is nearly 20-30% less than for the sitting posture.

If you stand up, rest for 5 minutes, and do the breath holding test (or body oxygen test) while standing, you will get smaller numbers. This is because your metabolism for the upright standing posture is about 20-30% higher. You require about 20-30% more oxygen and generate 20-30% more CO2. Therefore, your CP will be slightly shorter. For example, if your real CP while sitting is 20 seconds, then your standing CP will be about 15-16 seconds.

The same ideas about metabolism can be applied to the horizontal position. This means that our real CP numbers, when we wake up, are lower than the measured morning CP numbers. Therefore, the real overnight CP drop is greater than the decrease that is recorded in your daily log.

In practical terms, this indicates that, if you do not have any overnight CP losses, your morning CP should be slightly higher than your previous-evening CP.

Such situations (when the morning CP is greater than the evening CP) are very rare. In such cases, all these steps considered in this book are not essential. In fact, if your measured morning CP is higher than your last-evening CP, then you do not really need any major changes related to your sleep. Whatever you usually do in relation to sleep is fine, and you need to focus on how to increase your CP during the day.

This can be your goal: to make your morning CP greater than your evening CP. And the purpose of this book is to provide you with lifestyle changes and techniques to achieve this goal.

Our next step is to analyze which sleep-related factors make breathing heavier and reduce the morning CP.

1.10 Your morning CP: the key factor of your quality of sleep

There are two major rules that help us understand the role of the morning CP in one's health:

Rule #1: You need to make changes in your lifestyle and do something that relates to your sleep if your morning CP is significantly lower than your evening CP.

Rule #2: You can keep your sleep-related factors unchanged if your morning CP is very close to your evening CP.

Rule #1 suggests that, if your CP drops overnight, it is a sign and criteria for you need to to look for factors which can be improved. If you find these factors, you will be able to get higher morning CP numbers.

Rule #2 suggests that once your morning CP is nearly the same as your evening CP, then whatever factors you have right now, they are ok for you. In this case, you can focus on other factors that help you to achieve higher evening CP.

2. Which sleep factors cause health problems

In this chapter, we are going to explore those sleep factors and lifestyle parameters that increase breathing and cause lower morning CPs.

2.1 Sleeping too long

If a breathing student measures his or her CP during sleep, it can be observed that, for many people, for the first 4 hours of sleep, the CP is nearly the same. However, later, with each hour, there is a decline in the CP results. For many people, this large CP decrease takes place after 5 or 6 hours of sleep.

Severely sick people often experience a large CP drop either immediately after transition into any horizontal position or after only 1 or 2 hours of sleep. This is how Dr. Buteyko described this effect in his famous Lecture at the Moscow State University:

"Many severely sick patients remain sitting up, afraid to lie down. This is sensible. We should lie down only for a minimum amount of time, and only when sleeping. Our patients with deep breathing practice [breathing exercises], but cannot control their breathing at night, and hence, sleep is actually a poison for them. The longer he sleeps, the more chances that his breathing will be increased causing attacks."

However, with higher CPs, this problem becomes less severe. This is because people naturally sleep less when they have easier breathing during sleep and higher CPs. In fact, there is a Table that shows a correlation between breathing patterns and duration of sleep. It is provided below, in Chapter 4.

2.2 Wrong sleep positions

While most internet sources, including official medical websites, recommend sleeping on one's back (as the best sleep position), medical evidence (all 24 published studies) revealed worsening of the following health problems due to sleeping on one's back (supine sleep):
- Asthma (Ballard et al, 1991)
- Asthma and allergies in wheezing children (Ponsonby et al, 2004)
- Asthma (nocturnal) (D'Alonzo & Ciccolella, 1996)
- Back pain in pregnancy (Fast & Hertz, 1992)*
- Bruxism and swallowing (Miyawaki et al, 2003)
- Bruxism, clenching episodes and gastroesophageal reflux (Miyawaki et al, 2004)
- Chronic respiratory insufficiency patients (Ambrogio et al, 2009)
- Cough (nocturnal) and coughing attacks (Bonnet et al, 1995)
- GERD (gastroesophageal reflux disease) (Khoury et al, 1999; Wang et al, 1999)
- Geriatric inpatients (Hjalmarsen & Hykkerud, 2008)*
- Heart failure patients with central sleep apnea/Cheyne-Stokes (irregular) respiration (Joho et al, 2010; Szollosi et al, 2006*)
- Irregular or periodic breathing (Hudgel et al, 1993)
- Pregnancy (Trakada et al, 2003)*
- Sleep apnea (Ingman et al, 2004; Yoshida, 2000; Matsuzawa et al, 1995; Miura e tal, 1992; Kavey et al, 1985)
- Sleep paralysis and terrifying hallucinations (Kompanje, 2008; Cheyne, 2002)
- Snoring, hypopneas and apneas (Jan et al, 1994)
- Stroke patients with sleep apnea (Brown et al, 1998)
- Stroke (elderly patients) (Schubert & Héraud, 1994)
- Tuberculosis (pulmonary) treated by thoracoplasty (Brander et al, 1993)*

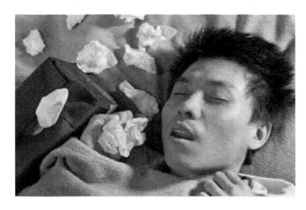

In several above-mentioned studies (see all references below) the researchers measured blood oxygen saturation. These studies are marked with the "*" sign above. It was found in all of them that the supine sleeping position produced the worst blood oxygenation in comparison with any other body posture (Fast & Hertz, 1992; Hjalmarsen & Hykkerud, 2008; Szollosi et al, 2006; Trakada et al, 2003; Brander et al, 1993).

References

Ambrogio C, Lowman X, Kuo M, Malo J, Prasad AR, Parthasarathy S, Sleep and non-invasive ventilation in patients with chronic respiratory insufficiency, Intensive Care Med. 2009 Feb;35(2):306-13. Epub 2008 Sep 16.

Ballard RD, Pak J, White DP, Influence of posture and sustained loss of lung volume on pulmonary function in awake asthmatic subjects, Am Rev Respir Dis. 1991 Sep;144(3 Pt 1):499-503.

Bonnet R, Jörres R, Downey R, Hein H, Magnussen H, Intractable cough associated with the supine body position. Effective therapy with nasal CPAP, Chest. 1995 Aug;108(2):581-5.

Brander PE, Salmi T, Partinen M, Sovijärvi AR, Nocturnal oxygen saturation and sleep quality in long-term survivors of thoracoplasty, Respiration. 1993;60(6):325-31.

Brown DL, Lisabeth LD, Zupancic MJ, Concannon M, Martin C, Chervin RD, High prevalence of supine sleep in ischemic stroke patients, Stroke. 2008 Sep;39(9):2511-4.

Cheyne JA, Situational factors affecting sleep paralysis and associated hallucinations: position and timing effects, J Sleep Res. 2002 Jun;11(2):169-77.

D'Alonzo GE, Ciccolella DE, Nocturnal asthma: physiologic determinants and current therapeutic approaches, Curr Opin Pulm Med. 1996 Jan;2(1):48-59.

Fast A, Hertz G, Nocturnal low back pain in pregnancy: polysomnographic correlates, Am J Reprod Immunol. 1992 Oct-Dec;28(3-4):251-3.

Hjalmarsen A, Hykkerud DL, Severe nocturnal hypoxaemia in geriatric inpatients, Age Ageing. 2008 Sep;37(5):526-9. Epub 2008 May 16.

Hudgel DW, Devadatta P, Hamilton H, Pattern of breathing and upper airway mechanics during wakefulness and sleep in healthy elderly humans, J Appl Physiol. 1993 May;74(5):2198-204.

Ingman T, Nieminen T, Hurmerinta K, Cephalometric comparison of pharyngeal changes in subjects with upper airway resistance syndrome or obstructive sleep apnea in upright and supine positions, Eur J Orthod. 2004 Jun;26(3):321-6.

Jan MA, Marshall I, Douglas NJ, Effect of posture on upper airway dimensions in normal human, Am J Respir Crit Care Med. 1994 Jan;149(1):145-8.

Joho S, Oda Y, Hirai T, Inoue H, Impact of sleeping position on central sleep apnea/Cheyne-Stokes respiration in patients with heart failure, Sleep Med. 2010 Feb;11(2):143-8.

Kavey NB, Blitzer A, Gidro-Frank S, Korstanje K, Sleeping position and sleep apnea syndrome, Am J Otolaryngol. 1985 Sep-Oct;6(5):373-7.

Khoury RM, Camacho-Lobato L, Katz PO, Mohiuddin MA, Castell DO, Influence of spontaneous sleep positions on nighttime recumbent reflux in patients with gastroesophageal reflux disease, Am J Gastroenterol. 1999 Aug;94(8):2069-73.

Kompanje EJ, 'The devil lay upon her and held her down'. Hypnagogic hallucinations and sleep paralysis described by the Dutch physician Isbrand van Diemerbroeck (1609-1674) in 1664, J Sleep Res. 2008 Dec;17(4):464-7.

Matsuzawa Y, Hayashi S, Yamaguchi S, Yoshikawa S, Okada K, Fujimoto K, Sekiguchi M, Effect of prone position on apnea severity in obstructive sleep apnea, Intern Med. 1995 Dec;34(12):1190-3.

Miura C, Hida W, Miki H, Kikuchi Y, Chonan T, Takishima T, Effects of posture on flow-volume curves during normocapnia and hypercapnia in patients with obstructive sleep apnea, Thorax. 1992 Jul;47(7):524-8.

Miyawaki S, Lavigne GJ, Pierre M, Guitard F, Montplaisir JY, Kato T, Association between sleep bruxism, swallowing-related laryngeal movement, and sleep positions, Sleep. 2003 Jun 15;26(4):461-5.

Miyawaki S, Tanimoto Y, Araki Y, Katayama A, Imai M, Takano-Yamamoto T, Relationships among nocturnal jaw muscle activities, decreased esophageal pH, and sleep positions, Am J Orthod Dentofacial Orthop. 2004 Nov;126(5):615-9.

Ponsonby AL, Dwyer T, Trevillian L, Kemp A, Cochrane J, Couper D, Carmichael A, The bedding environment, sleep position, and frequent wheeze in childhood, Pediatrics. 2004 May;113(5):1216-22.

Schubert V, Héraud J, The effects of pressure and shear on skin microcirculation in elderly stroke patients lying in supine or semi-recumbent positions, Age Ageing. 1994 Sep;23(5):405-10.

Szollosi I, Roebuck T, Thompson B, Naughton MT, Lateral sleeping position reduces severity of central sleep apnea / Cheyne-Stokes respiration, Sleep.2006 Aug 1;29(8):1045-51.

Trakada G, Tsapanos V, Spiropoulos K, Normal pregnancy and oxygenation during sleep, Eur J Obstet Gynecol Reprod Biol. 2003 Aug 15;109(2):128-32.

Wang Q, Liu J, Zhao X, Lei J, Cong Q, Li W, Li B, Wang F, Cao F, Zhang X, Zhang H, Zhang H, Can esophagogastric anastomosis prevent gastroesophageal reflux [Article in Chinese], Zhonghua Wai Ke Za Zhi. 1999 Feb;37(2):71-3, 3.

Yoshida K, The relationship between sleep position and therapeutic effect of the Esmarch-Scheine appliance in sleep apnea syndromes [Article in German], Fortschr Neurol Psychiatr. 2000 Feb;68(2):93-6.

2.3 Mouth breathing

If you have dry mouth and are thirsty when you wake up in the morning, it is nearly certain that you have been breathing through the mouth during sleep. For severely sick people and those people who suffer from rhinitis and related respiratory conditions, mouth breathing may take place as soon as they fall asleep. For other people, mouth breathing may appear only when they sleep on their back, but not for other sleep positions. Whatever the scenario, according to my approximate estimates, most people have mouth breathing during their sleep.

Some decades ago mouth breathing was socially abnormal and unacceptable. For example, one dictionary suggests that a "mouth-breather = n. a stupid person; a moron, dolt, imbecile". What are the confirmed mouth-breathing effects?

CO2-related biochemical effects of mouth breathing

CO_2 is not a toxic waste gas (see links to studies below). Research articles on respiration often mention such a physiological parameter known as dead space. It is about 150-200 ml in an average adult person: inside the nose, throat, and bronchi. This space helps to preserve additional CO_2 for the human body to invest elsewhere. During inhalations we take CO_2 enriched air from our dead space back into the alveoli of the lungs. When the mouth is used for respiration, the dead space volume decreases, since nasal passages are no longer a part of the breathing route. Consequently, air exchange is stronger if air goes directly from the outside air to the alveoli. This reduces alveolar O_2 and arterial blood CO_2 concentrations. Such an effect does not take place with nose breathing.

Furthermore, the nasal-breathing route provides more resistance for respiratory muscles as compared to oral breathing (the route for mouth breathing is shorter and it has a greater cross sectional area).

In their study "An assessment of nasal functions in control of breathing" (Tanaka et al, 1988), Japanese researchers discovered that end-tidal-CO_2 concentrations were higher during nose breathing than during oral breathing. This research study revealed that a group of healthy volunteers had an average CO_2 of about 43.7 mmHg for nose breathing and only around 40.6 mmHg for oral breathing. In practice, in terms of body oxygenation or the CP, this corresponds to 45 s and 37 s at sea level. Hence, mouth breathing reduces oxygenation of the whole body.

Each mouth breather needs to know this short summary of immediate negative biochemical effects of mouth breathing related to CO_2:

- Reduced CO_2 content in alveoli of the lungs (hypocapnia)

- Hypocapnic vasoconstriction (constrictions of blood vessels due to CO_2 deficiency causing reduced blood flow and O_2 delivery to all vital organs)

- The suppressed Bohr effect (which reduces O_2 release in tissues by red blood cells)

- Reduced oxygenation of cells and tissues of all vital organs of the human body

- Anxiety, stress, addictions, sleeping problems and negative emotions

- Slouching and muscular tension

- Biochemical stress due to cold, dry air entering into the lungs

- Biochemical stress due to dirty air (viruses, bacteria, toxic and harmful chemicals) entering the lungs

- Possible infections due to absence of the autoimmunization effect

- Pathological effects due to suppressed nitric oxide utilization, including vasoconstriction, decreased destruction of parasitic organisms, viruses, and malignant cells (by inactivating their respiratory chain enzymes) in alveoli of the lungs, inflammation in blood vessels, disruption of normal neurotransmission, hormonal effects.

Nose breathing delivers nitric oxide to lungs, blood and cells

Normal nose breathing helps us to use our own nitric oxide that is generated in the sinuses. The main roles of NO and its effects have been discovered quite recently (in the last 20 years). Three scientists even received a Nobel Prize for their discovery that a common drug, nitroglycerin (used by heart patients for almost a century), is transformed into nitric oxide. NO dilates blood vessels of heart patients, reducing their blood pressure and heart rate. Hence, they can survive a heart attack.

This substance or gas is produced in various body tissues, including the nasal passages. As a gas, it is routinely measured in exhaled air coming from the nasal passages. Therefore, we can't utilize our own nitric oxide, an important hormone, when we start mouth breathing.

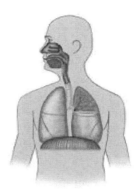

The confirmed functions of nitric oxide are:

- Destruction of viruses, parasitic organisms, and malignant cells in the airways and lungs by inactivating their respiratory chain enzymes.

- Regulation of binding/release of O_2 to hemoglobin. This effect is similar to the CO_2 function (the Bohr effect).

- Vasodilation of arteries and arterioles (regulation of blood flow or perfusion of tissues).

- Inhibitory effects of inflammation in blood vessels.

- Hormonal effects. NO influences secretion of hormones from several glands (adrenaline, pancreatic enzymes, and gonadotropin-releasing hormone).

- Neurotransmission. Memory, sleeping, learning, feeling pain, and many other processes are possible only with NO present (for transmission of neuronal signals).

Obviously, during mouth breathing, it is not possible to utilize one's own nitric oxide, which is produced in the sinuses. The mouth, according to Doctor Buteyko, is created by Nature for eating, drinking, and speaking. At all other times, it should be closed.

Cleaning, humidification and warming of air flow due to nose breathing

Our nasal passages are created to humidify, clean and warm the incoming flow of air due to the layers of protective mucus. This thin layer of mucus can trap about 98% to 99% of bacteria, viruses, dust particles, and other airborne objects.

If you are an endurance athlete and an asthmatic, you must train mostly, or even better, only, with nasal breathing. For really important competitions, you can use the mouth for breathing, but only if you have no current problems with your asthma. Sport training is useful due to its aerobic training effect. This is achievable while breathing only through the nose, as one Australian study confirmed (Morton et al, 1995; see the abstract in the references).

A group of US doctors from the Department of Surgery, University of Chicago even wrote an article with the title "Observations on the ability of the nose to warm and humidify inspired air". The abstract of their study is also provided in the references.

Mouth breathing influences on the autoimmunization effect

This is another advantage of nasal breathing over mouth breathing. The thin layer of mucus moves as a long carpet from sinuses, bronchi and other internal surfaces towards the stomach. Therefore, objects trapped by the mucus are discharged into the stomach, where GI enzymes and hydrochloric acid kill or weaken bacteria, viruses, fungi and other pathogens. Later, along the digestive conveyor, some of these pathogens (dead or weak) may leak from the small intestine into the blood (due to the intestinal permeability effect). Since these pathogens are either dead or weakened, they cannot do much harm (cannot cause infections). Moreover, they can provide a lesson for the immune system. This is exactly how natural auto-immunization can function successfully. Medical doctors and nurses inject vaccines with dead or weakened bacteria or viruses so as to teach and strengthen our immune response to these pathogens. Therefore, nasal breathing creates conditions for natural autoimmunization.

Practically speaking, when a household member is sick (as with a cold or flu), the still-healthy people could breathe either through their noses, teaching the own immune systems how to deal with the pathogenic bacteria or viruses. Or these household members can breathe through their mouths allowing these pathogens to gain access, settle and reproduce themselves in various parts of the body, causing infections.

Practical CP measurements suggest that mouth breathing significantly reduces body oxygenation during sleep, usually by about 30-70%, in some people nearly 2 times over. Also, keep in mind that effects of mouth breathing are accumulative, and the rate of accumulation is much higher than the rate related to longer sleep. In any case, just 20-30 min of mouth-breathing resets the breathing centre to lower CPs (body oxygen level), and such patients, as a rule, have less than 20 s for the morning body-oxygen test.

2.4 Electrical insulation from the Earth

At the present moment (2013), over 99% of people sleep ungrounded and remain ungrounded for the remaining part of the day. This means that their bodies are not electrically connected to the Earth. During nearly all of the evolution of the human species, we were connected to the Earth nearly all the time, due to our barefoot lifestyle. However, during the last century, due to the industrial revolution, humans started to use shoes made of rubber and other synthetic (i.e., nonconductive) materials.

When ungrounded, the human body has a tendency to accumulate a large positive electrical charge (i.e., a deficiency of free electrons), while grounding creates the same slightly negative charge as that of the Earth. Therefore, the Earth provides free electrons for the human body. Why could the electrical voltage of the human body be an important factor?

Numerous processes, such as the function of nerve and muscle cells, require a certain normal range of electrical voltages in the surrounding environment in order to work properly. Grounding (also called "Earthing") helps to normalize numerous processes. For example, grounding reduces blood viscosity due to its direct effects on clumping (aggregation) of red blood cells. It was discovered in a published study that red blood cells of ungrounded people cluster together due to a positive electrical body charge, while grounding immediately separates these clusters of cells, reducing blood viscosity and increasing blood flow. In conclusion, the authors wrote:

"Grounding increases the surface charge on RBCs and thereby reduces blood viscosity and clumping. Grounding appears to be one of the simplest and yet most profound interventions for helping reduce cardiovascular risk and cardiovascular events." (Chevalier et al, 2012)

It is clear that reduced blood viscosity helps to deliver more oxygen to body cells due to improved circulation.

There are some additional effects of free (unbonded) electrons. For example, free electrons are able to reduce (quench) inflammation and even prevent classical symptoms of inflammation, such as redness, swelling, pain, and immobility. In a clinical study conducted by Clint Ober (the man who discovered Earthing), 60 people tried grounding during sleep, and 93% of them reported improved quality of sleep, while 100% reported waking up feeling rested (Ober, 2000). Another study, titled "The biologic effects of grounding the human body during sleep as measured by cortisol levels and subjective reporting of sleep, pain, and stress", also found positive effects of grounding on sleep. This is a part of their abstract:

"Conclusions: Results indicate that grounding the human body to earth ("earthing") during sleep reduces night-time levels of cortisol and resynchronizes cortisol hormone secretion more in alignment with the natural 24-hour circadian rhythm profile. Changes were most apparent in females. Furthermore, subjective reporting indicates that grounding the human body to earth during sleep improves sleep and reduces pain and stress" (Ghaly & Teplitz, 2004).

There are many other studies that found positive effects of Earthing on normalization of numerous physiological functions and parameters in the human body.

References

Chevalier G, Sinatra ST, Oschman JL, Delany RM, Earthing (grounding) the human body reduces blood viscosity—a major factor in cardiovascular disease, J Altern Complement Med. 2012 Jul 3.

Ghaly M & Teplitz D, The biologic effects of grounding the human body during sleep as measured by cortisol levels and subjective reporting of sleep, pain, and stress, J Altern Complement Med. 2004 Oct;10(5):767-76.

Ober C, Grounding the human body to neutralize bioelectrical stress from static electricity and EMFs, ESD Journal, January, 2000.

2.5 The domino effect due to poor sleep

As we discussed above, when a person has a low morning CP due to hyperventilation during sleep, he or she produces physiological damage to the body. This includes damage to cells of the body, blood vessels, appearance of inflamed tissues, advance of pathogens, and many other effects. Depending on lifestyle, breathing exercises and physical activity, this damage gradually disappears. However, it takes many hours before this damage becomes negligible. What would you expect? How long does it take to eliminate all damage done by morning hyperventilation? In other words, what is the duration of physiological damage due to the overnight CP drop?

You have probably noticed that, if you wake up with a heavy head and feeling unhealthy due to poor quality of sleep and low morning CP, it will take you some hours before you feel better. Most people would say that they start to feel ok again only during late evening or night hours.

However, this effect is even more prolonged. It takes more than 24 hours to recover from the damage produced due to the Sleep Heavy Breathing Effect.

What does this mean practically? When you go to sleep, you still carry physiological damage from the previous night. As a result, since you do not control your breathing during sleep, this last-night damage intensifies your breathing again causing overbreathing and creating the foundation for poor next-night sleep. Therefore, it works like the domino effect.

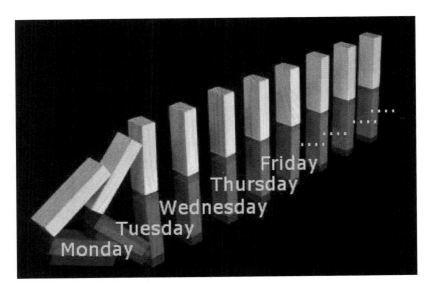

As you can see from this picture, if you have morning hyperventilation and a low CP on Monday, you are going to have poor sleep and a low morning CP on Tuesday. If you continue to have the same lifestyle, the following days of the week will bring you the same misery.

Note that the damage due to the overnight CP drop is present for people with a wide range of CPs. Some people have about 10 s for their usual daily CPs, and these people often suffer from this effect. However, those people who have about 35 s for the morning CP (their evening CPs can be up to 50-60 s) can also experience this domino effect related to poor sleep quality during consecutive nights.

This effect probably disappears at very high morning CPs of over 70-90 seconds. However, this domino effect takes place for nearly all sick and severely sick people (with less than 20 s for the morning CP), as well as for a vast majority of ordinary people.

Obviously, if you apply some special measures and manage to break, just for 2-3 nights, this vicious cycle related to your overnight CP drop, then you will be able to get much better sleep without changing other sleep parameters. In other words, if you stop 2 or 3 dominos in this chain reaction, then the remaining dominos will not fall. Then your future morning CPs will not be affected by overbreathing during the previous nights.

What does it take? Which methods will help to achieve this result? We are going to discuss these special methods later in this book.

2.6 Chest breathing

Chest (or thoracic) breathing is very common in modern people. When an adult person, especially a male, is asked to focus on their breathing, many of them start to breathe using the diaphragm. However, during sleep, most people are chest breathers.

Dr. Artour Rakhimov

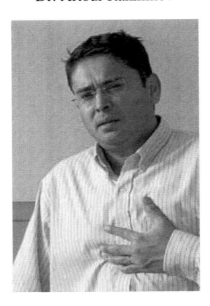

More than 90% of sick people have upper chest breathing during sleep. Chest breathing causes three fundamental health effects that promote chronic diseases and lead to low body-oxygen levels.

Chest breathing reduces blood oxygenation

The textbook *Respiratory Physiology* (West, 2000) suggests that the lower 10% of the lungs transports more than 40 ml of oxygen per minute, while the upper 10% of the lungs transports less than 6 ml of oxygen per minute. Hence, the lower parts of the lungs are about 6-7 times more effective in oxygen transport than the top of the lungs due to richer blood supply mostly caused by gravity.

During thoracic breathing, lower layers of the lungs, which are most valuable in oxygen transport, get much less, if any, fresh air (less oxygen supply). This causes reduced oxygenation of arterial blood in the lungs and can lead to so-called "ventilation-perfusion" mismatch (as in COPD or emphysema). Normal breathing is diaphragmatic, allowing homogeneous inflation of both lungs with fresh air, similar to what happens in the cylinder of a car engine due to the movement of the piston. Hence, during diaphragmatic breathing, all alveoli are homogeneously stretched vertically and get fresh air supply with higher O2 concentration for superior arterial blood oxygenation. In contrast, chest breathing creates problems with blood oxygenation. *This leads to reduced cell oxygenation: the driving force of all chronic diseases.*

This effect was discovered and, according to this study, is present in upright and sitting subjects. One may expect that any horizontal position would be better than sitting or standing due to reduced effects of gravity. Blood supply to the different parts of the lungs should be more homogeneous for any horizontal position.

However, as we discussed above, several clinical studies found significantly reduced blood oxygenation for supine sleep. It is not easy to explain this finding in terms of breathing mechanics, but it is likely that inhomogeneous blood and/or air supply to different parts of the lungs should play a leading role in this effect.

Chest breathing causes lymphatic stagnation

Dr. Shields, in his study "Lymph, lymph glands, and homeostasis" (Shields, 1992) reported that diaphragmatic breathing stimulates the cleansing work of the lymph system by creating a negative pressure pulling the lymph through the lymph system. This increases the rate of elimination of toxins from visceral organs by about 15 times. Why is this so?

The lymph system, unlike the cardiovascular system with the heart, has no pump. Lymph nodes are located in parts of the human body that get naturally compressed (squeezed) due to movements of body parts. For example, lymph nodes are located around the neck, above the armpits and in the groin area. Hence, when we move, stretch or turn the head, arms and legs, these lymph nodes get mechanical stimulation to push the lymph through valves. This is how the lymphatic system works. However, the lymph nodes connected to the stomach, kidneys, liver, pancreas, spleen, large and small intestines, and other vital organs are located just under the diaphragm - over 60% of all lymph nodes in total!

Hence, nature expects us to use the diaphragm in order to remove waste products from these vital organs all the time - literally with each breath, 24/7. Thus, chest breathing causes stagnation in the lymph system and accumulation of waste products in vital organs located under the diaphragm.

References

Shields JW, MD, *Lymph, lymph glands, and homeostasis*, Lymphology, Dec. 1992, 25, 4: 147.

West JB. *Respiratory physiology: the essentials*. 6th ed. Philadelphia: Lippincott, Williams and Wilkins; 2000.

2.7 Too warm conditions

Most people can confirm that they have experienced the effect related to sleeping in warm or very warm conditions, due to warm blankets, for example, while traveling or visiting their relatives or friends. Using too warm blankets prevents normal heat exchange. As a result, this causes intensified respiration.

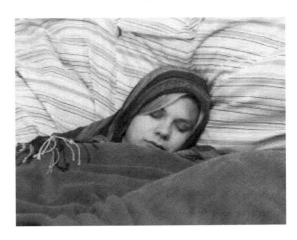

"An increase in temperature or overheating increases breathing not only in dogs, but in humans too."
Dr. Buteyko's Lecture at the Moscow State University.

2.8 Soft beds

Over 95% of people sleep on soft beds. Note that, according to the standards of Soviet and Russian Buteyko breathing doctors, even those mattresses that are called "hard" are still soft enough to cause hyperventilation, low body oxygenation, and poor health. When sleeping on a mattress, a person sleeps longer in the same position (often for many hours), while sleeping on a really hard bed (e.g., on the floor) feels uncomfortable, but produces a profound positive effect on the morning CP. Dr. Buteyko, in his Lecture, reported,

"Therefore we recommend to deep-breathing patients, especially children, to sleep on the tummy on a hard bed so that their spine is straight and not bent..."

3. Which other factors make sleep worse and reduce morning CP?

There are also influential sleep-affecting factors that are present during the day. First of all, any factor that makes your daily CP lower is going to have a negative effect on sleep. However, some of these factors have an additional negative effect on sleep. This chapter reviews some of these factors.

3.1 Late supper

Having a late meal, especially a big meal that requires over 2 hours for digestion, has an additional negative effect on sleep due to these 2 or more hours of hyperventilation during digestion. Even if you practice a breathing session after this meal and manage to increase your CP to your previous values, your breathing will be affected. This is because the breathing center remembers recent events, as in the domino effect considered above. Assume that you digest you meal from 9 to 11 pm, and then do the breathing session increasing your CP from 11:30 pm until midnight, when you go to sleep. On the one hand, your final CP can be close to your best numbers, but if you consider the last 3 hours (from 9 pm to midnight), you've had heavy breathing for more than 2 hours. Therefore, these 2 hours are going to produce a negative effect on your breathing during sleep.

If you eat your supper at about 5, 6 or 7 pm, then you will get much better CP profile during the last hours before sleep. As a result, your breathing during sleep will be lighter and slower.

3.2 A lack of physical exercise

When Dr. Buteyko and Soviet doctors are asked, "What is the main cause of hyperventilation in the modern population?" they say, "A lack of physical activity". These Soviet doctors studied thousands of their patients, after these patients completed their courses of breathing retraining, in order to find out **the long-term outcomes** of the Buteyko breathing method. Indeed, your long-term results are more important than your maximum CPs that you achieved during the breathing retraining course, and physical exercise is the most important single factor that defines one's long term success.

"Therefore, in relation to physical exercise or labor, there is a minimum standard for each person. If he exercises less, then he will die gradually. It is similar to a deficiency in vitamins, water, or food. We need about three hours of hard work every day to perspire. This will be a standard for man. He is made up of 60% muscles; these muscles must function. All joints must revolve in their entire amplitude. This is our intention and instruction."
Dr. Buteyko's Lecture at the Moscow State University.

An ability to incorporate reduced breathing into one's daily life is a very important parameter too.

Keep in mind that physical exercise, especially long sessions, does not produce an immediate positive effect on breathing and the CP (unless one uses the Training Mask - see http://www.normalbreathing.com/d/training-mask.php for more detail). The body needs time to adapt to the effects of physical exercise. The main positive effect of exercise is in the higher next-morning CP.

3.3 Nutritional deficiencies

Any nutritional deficiency, sooner or later, is going to make breathing heavier and the morning CP lower. You can find more details about nutritional deficiencies from a freely available manual "Major Nutrients Guide for Body O2: Ca, Mg, Zn and Fish Oil" posted on NormalBreathing.com.

A lack of essential fatty acids has a strong additional effect on overbreathing during sleep. Therefore, if you are low in essential fatty acids, you will have more problems with hyperventilation during sleep. Supplementation with fish oil or eating oily fish will increase your morning CP. Note that, for most people, vegetarian oils, such as hemp oil, flax seed oil, Udo oils and many others, are not able to solve this problem since their fatty acids are not converted into EPA and DHA. Therefore, for most people, especially with low CPs and/or digestive problems, these oils are useless.

Other nutritional deficiencies can worsen problems with sleep and cause lower morning CP.

3.4 A lack of cortisol

A deficiency in a natural hormone that is called "cortisol" also affects the morning CP. If a person has less than 20 s CP for many weeks or months, a gland that produces cortisol can get exhausted. Stress and inflammation are key factors that contribute to cortisol deficiency. As a result, some people are not able to increase their CPs, even when they practice long breathing sessions. It remains at about a 12-15 s CP level. This group of people often has less than 10 s for the morning CP due to a lack of cortisol.

Other people may be able to increase their CPs up to 18-25 s due to breathing exercises, but these individuals can still suffer from low morning CP due to insufficient blood cortisol levels. Depending on personal characteristics, there are various methods to solve this challenge.

3.5 Acute exacerbations

As we discussed above, overbreathing during sleep leads to the domino effect. A similar effect can take place due to acute exacerbations. This is because an acute attack causes a similar lasting impact on the human body. Any of these acute attacks during the day are going to influence sleep and cause lower morning CP:
- asthma attacks
- allergic reactions due to hay fever
- stroke
- heart attacks
- seizures due to epilepsy

- periods of critically low blood sugar (causing headaches)
- digestive flare-ups (e.g., due to Crohn's disease).

All these and many other exacerbations produce a lasting physiological stress that can include increased inflammation, generation of free radicals and other adverse effects. Therefore, it is crucial to avoid these attacks.

4. Blueprint of actions and first crucial steps

This Chapter is devoted to practical steps intended to directly counteract the negative effects of the sleep-related factors discussed in Chapters 2 and 3. We are going to consider the methods and techniques in the same order.

4.1 How to sleep less and better: the main goal

You are going to naturally sleep less when your CP gets higher and higher due to breathing retraining. Here is a table that provides the relationship between breathing parameters and quality/duration of sleep.

Duration and quality of sleep for different automatic breathing patterns			
Respiratory Frequency	Body oxygen test result	Duration of sleep	Quality of sleep
>26 breaths/min	<10 s	Often >10 hours	Often very poor
15-26 breaths/min	10-20 s	Often >9 hours	Often poor
12-20 breaths/min	20-40 s	6-8 hours	Insomnia possible
7-12 breaths/min	40-80 s	4 hours	Excellent
5 breaths/min	2 min	3 hours	Excellent
3 breaths/min	3 min	2 hours	Excellent

Of course, the main problem here is that it may take some weeks or even months before you get up to 40+ s for your morning CP, when you have a great quality of sleep and these 4 hours of sleep do not make your CP lower. Therefore, the table provides your long-term goal.

There are also additional steps you can take to directly reduce the duration of your sleep. Let me start with Dr. Buteyko's introduction:

"Our patients with deep breathing practice [breathing exercises], but cannot control their breathing at night, and hence, sleep is actually a poison for them. The longer he sleeps, the more chances that his breathing will be increased causing attacks. Therefore, we wake him up after 1-2 hours, he practices decreasing respiration, we reduce his sleep down to 4-5 hours in a 24-hour period, not more, and he cures himself. Later, when the breathing is corrected, sleep becomes less than the norm. It reduces itself. It gets deeper and deeper. This alarms many patients, "Previously, I was sleeping for 8 hours and it was not enough, but now I sleep 4 hours and get enough". Yes, it is possible to get enough sleep in 4 hours with very light breathing." Dr. Buteyko's Lecture at the Moscow State University.

When your morning CP is less than 40 seconds, restriction of sleep to only 4-5 hours can be a challenge. As you can imagine, when breathing students try this method, they usually feel sleepy during the day. The solution to this problem is to have short naps, about 5-10 minutes long, during the day. If you find it too hard, you can either extend your night sleep up to about 6 hours and/or have a longer nap in the afternoon.

4.2 Best sleep positions

In relation to the best sleep positions, these Soviet and Russian Buteyko doctors, while testing thousands of their patients, found that there is the following approximate relationship between sleeping postures and the body-oxygen level or the results for the CP test:

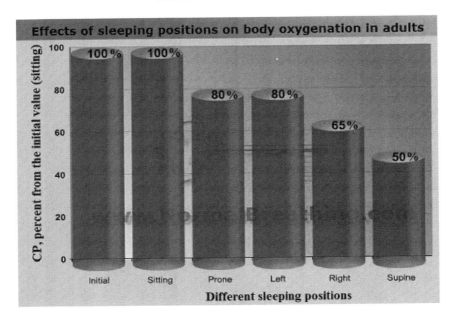

Prone position: lying with the front or face downward. **Supine position:** lying down with the face up.

Sitting posture for sleep

Sitting (as in an armchair or bus/plane seat) is the ideal-sleeping posture for breathing and body oxygenation. Russian Buteyko doctors have the same opinion (e.g., Chief Physician of the Moscow Buteyko Clinic Andrey Novozhilov, private communication). Honorable physician and doctor-therapist of the Moscow Buteyko Clinic, Tatiana Alexandrovna Kulik, in her book "Buteyko Method for All" (ISBN: 978-5-9731-0213-5; Moscow, ASS-Centre; 2010, 124 pages, in Russian) also states that sitting is the ideal posture for sleep.

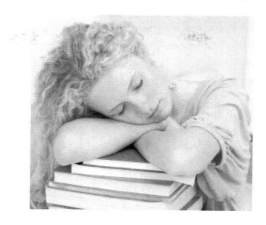

Unfortunately, since modern people do not learn how to sleep sitting from early childhood, most of them find it uncomfortable. However, it is very efficient for speedy breathing normalization and can be applied in special circumstances provided that the angle of body inclination remains high.

This position allows much easier transition to the over-40-s morning-CP health zone. This transition and your adaptation to sleeping sitting will be much easier if you follow these suggestions and requirements:

- Make sure that you have **solid support for your elbows**. If elbows are hanging in air, it creates additional pressure on shoulders and makes sleeping sitting harder.

- Provide **a support for your neck using a travel pillow**. Since nearly all outer cases of travel pillows are made of artificial or synthetic fabrics, you can make a travel pillow from a towel.

- In addition, it is good to have **a support for the back of your head** during sleep. Preferably, this support should be soft, as in long-distance buses and planes.

- Make sure that **your body trunk is nearly vertical or at 80-90 degrees to the horizon**. Inclined or reclined sleep positions are nearly as bad for health and breathing as supine sleep.

Some people are able to easily adapt to sleeping sitting with great health benefits due to the morning CP miracle effect. The CP does not drop! Other people can find it uncomfortable, but they can still go on and sleep sitting for several nights in a row. Even if you are not able to get used to this sleeping posture for good, you still can get great benefits while using this posture for 2 or 3 consecutive nights. This can be done in order to eliminate the domino effect described above or to break through 40 s morning CP threshold.

Once the desirable result is achieved, there is no need to continue to sleep sitting. However, if you are able to adapt to sleep in a sitting position for many days or weeks, you will get a large advantage in comparison with many other people.

Horizontal sleep positions

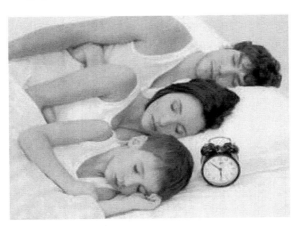

If you found the sitting sleeping position too uncomfortable, you need to alternate between the 2 best horizontal positions: sleeping on your stomach (or chest) and the left side. Note that there are many intermediate positions between chest and left or right side. If you prop one of your shoulders with a pillow, you can sleep half-way on your chest and this position is also good for maintaining light and slow breathing and good body oxygenation.

If you are forced to sleep on your back

There is a small group of people, with severe back pain, IBD during recent exacerbations, and some other health problems, who can only sleep in the supine position. In order to prevent overbreathing during sleep, these people should use mechanical restriction of ventilation ("swaddling of adults"). This method is described below.

You can measure the effects of sleeping positions on your body oxygen

If you are uncertain about the suggested ideas, you can measure changes in your CP after sleeping in different positions for 10 or more minutes. In order to do that, keep an illuminated electronic clock or ticking clock nearby for counting your CP at night. Then you do not need to turn the light on. If you find that your CP remains the same or even gets higher after sleeping in certain positions, it is smart to use them for improving your health and ignore these and any other statistical findings. However, such situations are exceptionally rare.

Chapters 6 and 7 provide additional details related to optimum sleep positions.

4.3 How to ensure nose breathing

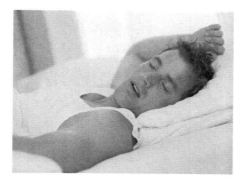

In the 1960s, in order to ensure nasal breathing and stop mouth breathing during the night, Russian patients invented **mouth taping**, which is now a part of the Buteyko breathing method. There are also other methods that do not require a tape. All these techniques are described below.

How to tape one's mouth at night to stop mouth breathing

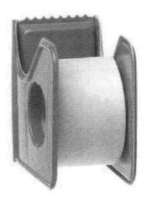

For mouth taping one needs a surgical tape and cream to prevent the tape from sticking to lips. Both can be bought in the pharmacy. Micropore (or 3M) and vaseline are popular choices. First, put a small amount of cream on the lips so that it is easy to remove the tape in the morning. Then take a small piece of tape and stick it in the middle, vertically, across the closed mouth. Some students prefer to put it along or horizontally, but a small piece in the middle is sufficient. If you are afraid to seal the mouth completely, tape only one half of the mouth leaving space for emergency breathing.

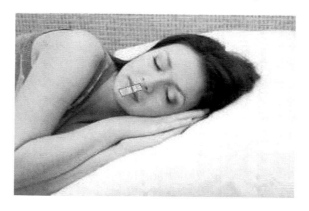

In 2006 one of my Buteyko method colleagues, Dr. James Oliver, a GP from the UK and former president of the Buteyko Breathing Association made a presentation to the British Thoracic Society about the safety of mouth taping based on thousands of cases both in Russia and in the west. Previously he conducted a survey of Buteyko method teachers and obtained the statistical data.

Mouth taping at night to stop mouth breathing should normally be a temporary measure. When one's CP (body oxygen level) is above 20 s in the morning, mouth taping is no longer necessary.

Can mouth taping create distress?

A majority of students have no problems with mouth taping and they breathe only through the nose during the whole night. Their mouth is not dry in the morning and they report numerous benefits of mouth taping.

However, some students may find it difficult and uncomfortable so that they remove the tape during the night. These incidents have physiological causes, including:

1. Sleeping on the back

If you turn on your back during night sleep, your breathing gets almost twice as heavy, and it will be very difficult to pump more air through the nose. Hence, learn the module devoted to prevention of sleeping on one's back.

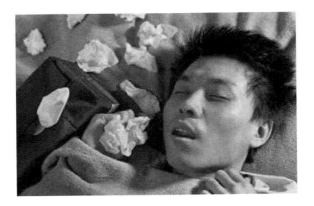

2. Overly warm sleep conditions

If your blanket is too warm, your breathing becomes deeper during sleep. You will wake up because heavy breathing through the nose is uncomfortable. To prevent overheating, use less warm clothes and blankets during sleep.

3. Carpets in your bedroom

Presence of carpets makes air quality tens or even hundreds of times worse. During night sleep several cubic meters of air with millions of airborne particles, including dust, dust mites, their droppings, bacteria, viruses, paint, fire retardants, and other chemicals will enter through the nasal passages. This makes the nose dryer. Airborne particles cause stress for the immune system and lead to deeper breathing. Sleeping in carpet-free rooms or covering carpets with plastic will solve this problem.

4. Dusty pillow cases, blankets, and bed sheets.

They create the same effect as carpets. There are other sources of dust such as books, newspapers, hanging clothes, and old dusty curtains. Make sure that your bedroom has good air quality.

5. Closed windows during the night

This factor greatly worsens air quality in the bedroom due to poor air circulation and absence of air ions that make air cleaner. Either keep windows open or, if it is too cold or too noisy outside, buy an air ionizer/purifier and keep it running through the night.

6. Skin rashes and allergic reactions due to skin sensitivity

Try to find a hypoallergic tape or surgical paper tape. If rashes and allergic reactions are still a problem, you can apply the alternative solutions provided below.

Alternatives to mouth taping

1. You can tape around your mouth as it is shown on the picture below (but do not use the same sleeping posture unless you have severe back pain or other serious reasons).

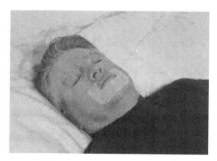

**Taping around
the mouth**

2. Sew together two clean socks making a circle. Wear it at night around your head so that to keep your jaw closed.

3. Buy chin straps that are promoted for people with sleep apnea or snoring. They can be ordered online and cost from about $5 up to $30 USD.

4.4 How to ground yourself

You can ground yourself (get electrically connected with Earth) for some part of the day, for better sleep, and/or during sleep using simple techniques and/or objects discussed on this page. Most people are able to find nearly all required materials and parts to create grounding devices in their own household. Many grounding methods do not require any special objects.

Note that the soles of feet and arms are the most conductive areas on the surface of the human body.

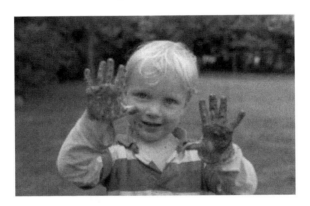

Warning. Excessive grounding (for previously ungrounded and currently sick people or pregnant females) can trigger a cleansing reaction and is potentially very dangerous. Therefore, as for breathing retraining, grounding yourself requires a good knowledge of temporary restrictions and contraindications. These details are provided on NormalBreathing.com.

How to ground yourself during daytime

1. Barefoot walking or barefoot running can be the easiest and cheapest option. If you are new to barefoot activities, use this method for some weeks only in the first part of the day (before 6 pm or even 2 pm) since excessive stimulation of nerve endings of the feet can cause problems with sleep.

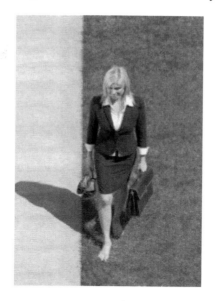

If you can find soft grass, a good barefoot grounding session requires about 30 minutes. However, if you have not done barefoot walking for some weeks or longer, 30 min can be too invigorating for the nervous system. Many people get problems with sleep due to excessive sympathetic stimulation. Even 5 minutes of barefoot walking before sleep can cause problems. Therefore, if you are new to barefoot walking, start with about 10 min, better in the early morning (wet grass is more conductive), but remain connected with the Earth for another 20 minutes, while doing, for example, stretching and/or other exercises that do not cause significant additional stimulation of your feet. You can increase the duration of barefoot walking gradually, by about 2 min on each consecutive day until you get about 30 minutes per session.

For people with moderate and severe forms of diseases, especially inflammatory conditions, it is suggested to have about 1 hour of barefoot connection per day. Later, with a higher morning CP, you will need less grounding. Therefore, you may wish to have another session of barefoot grounding on the same day.

However, during initial stages, do not use barefoot walking within 6 hours before sleep, and keep in mind the importance of restrictions for intensity and duration of feet stimulation. Different surfaces produce variable effects. For example, walking for 1 minute on pebbles causes about the same stimulation as walking for 10 minutes on soft grass. Therefore, for a novice, even 1 minutes of intensive stimulation due to barefoot walking can prevent him or her from sleeping for several hours.

Barefoot walking is most effective when it is done on the coast of the ocean or sea provided that your feet are in contact with sea water. This is a very powerful technique since sea water is an exceptionally good conductor.

2. You can ground yourself using a simple device that is shown on the right. This particular homemade DIY device can be used only in the USA and Canada since it is made for a three prong US outlet. If you are located in a different country, study the details provided below.

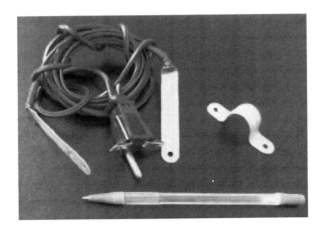

In order to make this device, you need:
- an electrical cable
- 2 copper clad clamps (which can be found in hardware stores)
- a standard three prong plug
- electrical tape.

You can get electrically connected (or grounded) with Earth using a copper cable, which is easy to find in electrical and hardware stores. (Other electrical cables can be used too.)

Both electrodes (copper pieces of this device) can be kept on the soles of your feet (barefoot, or in your socks, or sandals) or on your waist (less preferable due to much better conductivity of soles).

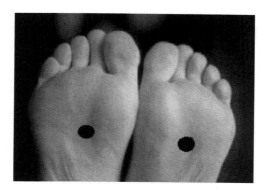

The pieces of copper can be attached to your K1 (Kidney 1) acupuncture points (see the picture), which are probably the most conductive places on the skin of the body. You can fix those flat copper pieces on the K1 points using a surgical tape for better connection. Several studies used these acupuncture points for Earthing of their subjects.

This is one of the simplest and cheapest methods to start with. If you use a plug with a cable from old electrical appliances, keep in mind that the ground wire is located in the middle.

As you can see on the picture of the device, 2 upper prongs (flat prongs) of the plug are bent for safety reasons, while the round prong (for grounding) is left for use.

3. **Foot bath with salty water.** In your home, fill a wide foot basket with 2-3 liters of water. Add 2-3 tablespoons of sea salt and stir to dissolve. Keep one or both copper electrodes in water, with another end of the cable connected to Earth. If there are no contraindications,

use it 2, 3 or more times per day. This last method provides nearly an ideal connection between Earth and the human body and provides the best grounding for feet.

How to ground yourself during sleep

Earthing during sleep is the suggested method especially for those people who have low results for the morning body-oxygenation test. One end of the grounding cable should be connected to Earth and the other one to an object that will be in contact with your body.

Where to attach the grounding end?

There are different options for grounding depending on your current location and availability of plumbing and heating tubes.

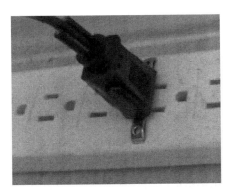

1. If your sockets are connected with a ground (Earth) cable, this is the cable that you can get connected to. The solution **for the USA and Canada** was mentioned above. Here is an image of such a plug attached to a ground cable of a socket (the left picture).

2. If you are located in **the UK or Ireland**, you can disassemble the plug (usually you need to unscrew one or more bolts), and get connected only with the upper middle prong connected to Earth. You can do the same in other countries that have ground cables connected to Earth.

3. You can also get connected to plumbing or central heating tubes (see the image). In this image, the copper part of the cable was separated from a plastic coating (this can be done with ordinary scissors), and then this end was fixed with electrical tape.

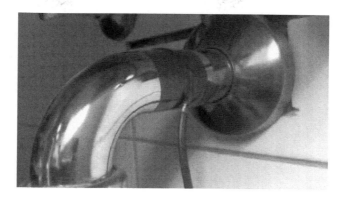

Other types of tape may also be used. The crucial thing is to achieve good contact between the metal parts. Ideally, you need to wind the metal wires around the tube at least 1 or 2 times. Also, make sure that your cable is attached to pure metal that does not have paint on it since generally paints are nonconductive.

Devices and electrodes for body contact

1. A simple DIY device (see the picture above) with 2 copper pieces can be used to get connected with Earth during sleep. You can wear socks during sleep and keep the device electrodes in socks. Optionally, you can use a surgical tape for keeping the copper pieces attached to K1 points.

2. It is possible to apply **a conductive tape** on your bed linen and get a strip across the bed so that your body has contact with this metal strip during sleep. However, such conductive tapes can be found only in special electrical stores. Here is a similar solution how to ground yourself using materials that can be found in many homes.

If you have (or can find) an ordinary aluminum foil (used for baking) and a wide plastic tape (or duct tape, or blue tape),

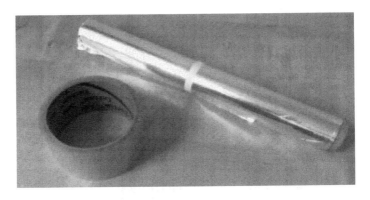

then you can easily make a grounding metal strip from these materials. How? Attach about 50-60 cm (20-24 inches) of aluminum foil to the sticky side of the tape. Then you need to fix this metal strip in the middle of your bed. The next image shows this metal strip located on a bed sheet.

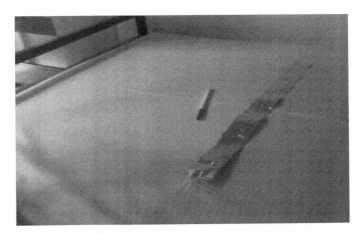

Warning. *Make sure that the uncovered metal part is facing up so that your body can touch it during sleep and you can get grounded yourself. If you sleep on the side that is covered with plastic, you may be poorly grounded or not grounded at all.*

Warning. *Avoid using foils from potato chips and similar food wrappings. Both sides of such foils are usually covered with a thin (invisible) layer of plastic that prevents electrical current and flow of electrons. At least, if you use them, check that your foil is conductive.*

After this, you should connect this metal strip with the end of the copper wire. You can achieve this using a simple scotch-type tape or an electrical tape.

There are many other ways to ground yourself. Which methods are better? One of the effects of grounding is that generally sick and severely sick people have stronger perspiration with higher conductivity of their skin. As a result, they get more electrons during grounding.

Regarding the methods themselves, their efficiency depends on:
- surface area of grounding
- skin conductivity of this area (or resistance)
- duration of grounding.

Warning. *Do not use grounding during thunderstorms due to presence of lightning. In the long run, personal safety can be increased with application of resistors and blow-up fuses to prevent even miniscule chances of electrocution.*

Other methods to ground yourself

If you find Earthing beneficial, you can either investigate more on this topic or purchase Earthing products online. You can buy the Earthing mat (about $60 USD, as of August 2013), Earthing half sheet (about $170 USD), or Fitted Earthing Sheets (for $230 USD) made of cotton and fine silver wires threaded in, for conductivity.

4.5 Eliminating the domino effect

In order to break the vicious circle of morning hyperventilation so that you do not hyperventilate during the next night, you can apply 2 main techniques. The first technique is called **the wake-up method**.

The wake-up method

This method was created in the 1960's by Dr. Buteyko for severely sick and critically ill people. As he found, these groups of people have serious problems with overbreathing during sleep. We discussed above that, for most people, their sleep is relatively good for up to 5-6 hours, but later they start to hyperventilate. In severely sick and hospitalized people, additional overbreathing (on top of existing chronic hyperventilation) takes place sooner, sometimes only after 1-2 hours of sleep or even immediately after the transition into a horizontal position.

The idea of the method is simple. The person needs to wake up before the onset of additional hyperventilation, do breathing exercises and, possibly, some light physical activity, and then can go to sleep again.

"Many severely sick patients remain sitting up, afraid to lie down. This is sensible. We should lie down only for a minimum amount of time, and only when sleeping. Our patients with deep breathing practice [breathing exercises], but cannot control their breathing at night, and hence, sleep is actually a poison for them... The longer he sleeps, the more chances that his breathing will be increased causing attacks. Therefore, we wake him up after 1-2 hours, he practices decreasing respiration ..."
Dr. Buteyko's Lecture at the Moscow State University.

For people with low body weight and problems with hypoglycemia (low blood glucose)

Note that people with low body weight and problems with hypoglycemia (low blood glucose) may require a small snack, after this breathing session, in order to fall asleep again. These groups of people then should have an additional breathing session after the meal is digested. Or they can have a suitable soft and smooth snack (such as raw honey, fruit juices, and so forth) before doing the breathing session. Most people, however, could be feeling slightly hungry, but they do not require eating in order to fall asleep and have good sleep later.

Here are some general ideas related to the wake up method applied to different groups of people.

For severely sick people with a morning CP of about 10 s or less

For example, imagine a severely sick person who can safely sleep for only 2 hours. Then he starts to hyperventilate with a good chance of having attacks or acute episodes. To avoid acute exacerbations, he can set an alarm in order to wake up after 1.5-2 hours of sleep. After waking up, he needs to do a breathing session for at least 12, better up to 20 min long. (Breathing devices would be nearly 2 times more effective). For these breathing exercises, he needs to sit down, with his feet on the floor. In other words, these breathing sessions cannot be done while lying in the bed, in the horizontal position. This breathing session, in the middle of the night, will help him to sleep without hyperventilation for the next 2 hours. Then he again should wake up and do his breathing exercises.

Severely sick people may need to wake up up to 3-4 or even more times in order to avoid acute episodes during sleep and to create conditions for better sleep. Therefore, while these steps can be quite hard to implement, he does not need to do them every night. This method can be applied for only 2-3 nights. Later, the duration of his good sleep (i.e., without overbreathing and CP drop) will likely be much longer, possibly up to 4-5 hours or more. Therefore, he can later have only one wake up throughout the night.

For people with higher CPs (15+ s)

If you have a higher CP (e.g., about 15-20 s in the morning), you will also benefit from having one wake up after about 4 hours of sleep. In this case of only one wake-up, your quality of sleep and wellbeing in the morning are greatly improved due to the breathing session in the middle of the night. We can compare 2 scenarios:

1. In usual conditions, your breathing gets heavy after about 4-5 hours of sleep. As a result of overbreathing during the second half of

your sleep, your health is compromised and damage to organs and cells is done. Therefore, you will feel miserable in the morning.

2. When you have a breathing session after about 4 hours of sleep, your breathing pattern and quality of sleep during the second part of the night are much better. Therefore, while it can be challenging to do the breathing session in the middle of the night, your next morning wellbeing outweighs the small temporary disadvantages of waking up during sleep.

Obviously, this is a great technique to deal with the domino effect related to next-morning hyperventilation. This method, with one wake up during the night, works in a wide range of CPs. You can have:

- the overnight CP drop from about 15 down to 8-10 seconds, as in most sick people with moderate forms of heart disease, asthma, bronchitis, epilepsy, cancer, and many other conditions

- the overnight CP drop from about 25 down to about 15 seconds, as in most ordinary people who do not suffer from serious illnesses but still have lousy health

- the overnight CP drop from about 35 down to about 25 seconds, as in relatively healthy people

- or the overnight CP drop from about 45-50 or more down to about 35 seconds, as in advanced breathing students.

In all these situations, this method will allow you to significantly increase your morning CP.

Once you have higher morning CP, you need to get stabilized in your new zone in the Buteyko Table of Health Zones using other methods so that you do not need to wake up at night every single night for the rest of your life. In order to keep your higher morning CPs, most people need to increase the duration and intensity of their physical exercise. Keep in mind that, at higher morning CPs, it is much easier to exercise. In fact, nearly all people notice a greatly increased natural desire to do more exercise. Also, higher morning CPs will create conditions for your further progress in final CPs after breathing exercises. As a result, you will also likely get record numbers for your final CPs. This is an additional stimulus for improved overall progress and greatly enhanced health.

The swaddling technique

Apart from the wake up method, in order to eliminate hyperventilation during sleep, Dr. Buteyko and other Soviet doctors developed and tested the technique that they called "mechanical restrictions of ventilation". It is sometimes called "swaddling of adults".

This method, according to the practice of Russian doctors, can be used for one of the three reasons (Souliagin, 1991):

- the initial stages of the breathing retraining (to have a faster increase in one's CP)

- temporary critical states

- the cleansing reactions.

The goal of this technique is to prevent deep breathing, and, more specifically, to reduce the contribution of chest breathing and amplitude of inspiration (the same as during breathing exercises with a use of a belt, as we discussed above), while preserving quiet relaxed exhalation.

You can find detailed instructions for three types of swaddling methods in Chapter 6 of this book.

4.6 Chest breathing

Chest breathing during sleep can be prevented using the swaddling methods that are described below. Note that chest breathing develops due to overbreathing, and it disappears at higher CPs, usually when one has more than 30 seconds for the morning CP. Therefore, technically speaking, prevention of chest breathing during sleep is a problem mainly of those people who have over 30 s CP during the day, and less than 30 s for the morning CP.

People with lower CPs (less than 30 s during the day) usually suffer from chest breathing 24/7. However, during sleep, their chest breathing becomes heavier. Therefore, they also suffer from chest overbreathing during sleep.

4.7 Too warm conditions

Thermoregulation during sleep can cause serious problems with overbreathing if someone has blankets and/or environmental conditions that are too warm. For most people, especially the overweight, the optimum strategy is to feel as cold as possible, while still able to fall asleep. If you wake up during sleep thinking, "It seems quite cold, but not too cold", and you are still able to fall asleep in seconds, this is about an ideal scenario for thermoregulation during sleep.

However, there are some exceptions. Underweight people, due to their low or borderline low blood glucose levels, often have much worse quality of sleep or even are not able to fall asleep if they are just a little bit cold. They need to keep themselves comfortably warm during sleep. People with respiratory infections and those who have less than 20 s for their daily CP numbers also require warm conditions during sleep.

Therefore, we can see again here that conventional understanding and acceptance of comfort are factors that destroy health during sleep. Many modern people, often with the background in health care, suggest and teach to people that we require:

- supine sleep, as the most comfortable sleep position

- warm blankets for feeling warm and comfortable

- soft beds, also for the reasons of comfort.

All these factors are accepted as healthy by millions of people. However, scientific evidence and practical experience related to hundreds of thousands of people suggest the opposite scenario. Now we can turn attention to the last remaining factor: softness of beds.

4.8 Soft beds

When someone says "I sleep on a hard bed", they usually imply that they sleep on a mattress that is harder than most other mattresses. However, as Soviet Buteyko doctors found in thousands of their patients, these mattresses are not hard enough for optimum sleep and the highest possible morning CP. If your CP drops during sleep, you definitely need to try, at least for 3 nights in row, sleeping on a really hard surface. By a "really hard surface", I mean sleeping on a floor or a piece of wood, such as plywood or a bench.

Can you have any materials and fabrics on the floor or the surface you sleep on? If you sleep on the carpet, you may have one layer of a bed linen. If you sleep on a wooden surface, you can use a very large towel or a thin blanket covered with a bed linen. If you sleep in a pajama suit, you can sleep directly on a carpet or a wooden surface.

One of the greatest obstacles to great or normal health is an emotional attachment of a person to various material gimmicks and useless things, such as soft warm beds, that destroy human health. Therefore, for most people, the idea of sleeping on a really hard surface generates pathetic feelings of a horrible loss. Their imagination produces pictures of self-suffering and excessive restrain. Strangely enough, many people do not realize that their usual day-after-day existence is an example of chronic misery, suffering, and pain.

Even people without an overnight CP drop are likely to get health benefits from sleeping on hard beds.

4.9 Sleep restriction

Apart from all these methods that lead to shorter sleep naturally, Dr. Buteyko and his medical colleagues also discovered that their patients achieve health improvements and higher morning CPs faster if these patients deliberately restrict their sleep to about 6 hours per night. In order to get a clearer picture, here is one of the Dr. Buteyko's quotes about sleep restriction and use of breathing exercises at night.

"Many severely sick patients remain sitting up, afraid to lie down. This is sensible. We should lie down only for a minimum amount of time, and only when sleeping. Our patients with deep breathing practice [breathing exercises], but cannot control their breathing at night, and hence, sleep is actually a poison for them... The longer he sleeps, the more chances that his breathing will be increased causing attacks. Therefore, we wake him up after 1-2 hours, he practices decreasing respiration, we reduce his sleep down to 4-5 hours in a 24-hour period, not more, and he cures himself. Later, when the breathing is corrected, sleep becomes less than the norm. It reduces itself. It gets deeper and deeper. This alarms many patients, "Previously, I was sleeping for 8 hours and it was not enough, but now I sleep 4 hours and get enough". Yes, it is possible to get enough sleep in 4 hours with very light breathing."
Dr. Buteyko's Lecture at the Moscow State University.

Let us consider the main benefits of sleep restriction using an example:

Imagine a person with a moderate degree of some chronic disease, with about 15 seconds for daily CP numbers and about 10-12 seconds for the morning CP. This person sleeps for about 8 hours per night. It is common for such people with moderate forms of diseases to experience a transition to heavier breathing after about 4-5 hours of sleep or at about 4 am. This means that he destroys his health during the remaining part of sleep or the last 3-4 hours. The damage due to overbreathing during sleep is proportional to the duration of this period of acute hyperventilation.

Now assume that this person restricts his sleep from 8 hours down to 6 hours. As a result of shorter sleep, the duration of his hyperventilation, with damage to body cells and organs, drops from 3-4 hours down to 1-2 hours. This is a very significant improvement. He will be able to greatly accelerate his overall CP growth, probably about 2 times or more.

If the same person, in addition, applies the wake-up method with one breathing session after 3-4 hours of sleep, he can completely eliminate overbreathing during sleep.

Depending on individual factors, most people are able to cut their night's sleep down to about 6 hours without negative effects on quality of life and daily performance. In fact, due to fast increase in their morning CPs, their quality of life and daily performance are going to be improved.

Important note about daytime naps

It is common for many people who use sleep restriction to experience periods of excessive yawning with a strong desire to sleep during afternoon hours, or from about noon up to 5-6 pm. During these periods of sleepiness, it is beneficial to take a short nap for about 5-10 minutes. If sleep restriction at night was not too excessive, a person will wake up naturally in 5-10 minutes feeling refreshed and with no desire to sleep more. However, it is important to take these naps while in a sitting position, in an armchair or couch. Naps in a horizontal position, during daytime, often produce some negative effects on wellbeing and should be avoided.

Three levels of sleep restriction

In order to have more clarity, I will describe 3 levels of sleep restriction. Note that individual requirements in sleep can be very different. There are many people who can sleep for 4-5 hours naturally, even while having only about 10 s CP and with no complaints about not enough sleep. However, in order to have some general guidance, here are some details about the common practice of Soviet doctors.

Level 1: Severe sleep restriction (down to 4-5 hours)

This method was applied by Dr. Buteyko and his numerous colleagues on thousands of severely sick people, often hospitalized, with various health problems. It is combined with breathing sessions after 1-2 hours of sleep, as it follows from the above quote from Dr. Buteyko's Lecture. People with severe sleep restriction may need up to 2-3 naps during day or may even fall asleep for about 1 hour or more. Depending on personal circumstances (including recent meals, current CP and physical exercise), long sleep during daytime can be safe since it is done in a sitting position.

I consider severe sleep restriction as an excellent temporary technique that can be used by severely sick and critically ill people in order to achieve a quick CP boost and to get to a safer zone with 15+ s or even 20+ s for their morning CPs. However, if you apply this technique for a longer time, you will get even higher morning CP numbers.

When the personal CP is higher (and the motivational factor to survive disappears), this technique of severe sleep restriction requires strict self-discipline. As a result, it can be used for a longer time only by people with strong will power and/or a natural ability to tolerate short sleep well.

Those people who have a strong will power and willing to try the application of the original Buteyko method in relation to sleep restriction can try to restrict their sleep to 4-5 hours.

Level 2: Moderate sleep restriction (down to 6 hours)

This is a relatively easy technique that can be safely and effectively used by most people. It often results in light daytime sleepiness, which is easy to tolerate. One nap in the afternoon (5-10 minutes is usually enough) greatly replenishes personal energy levels. You can

90

apply this method when you have nearly any morning CPs: about 10, or 15, or 20-25 seconds. With over 30 s for the morning CP, people wake up naturally after 6 hours of sleep. In addition, at 30+ s MCP, breathing students generally do not experience any sleepiness during daytime and do not require a daily nap.

If you find out during the day that 6 hours of sleep is too little for you, you can try to "survive" with 7 hours of sleep. It is still enough to get benefits from this method since the purpose of the technique is to increase your morning CP and/or to break the domino effect related to low morning CPs on consecutive days.

Level 3: Light sleep restriction (down to 7 hours)

This is a very easy method for nearly all people. With a breathing session at night, this technique also allows fast overall CP progress. Natural reduction of sleep down to 7 hours often occurs when the morning CP is over 20 seconds. With a slightly higher morning CP (30+ s), sleep will be even shorter naturally.

Note that since some people naturally have shorter sleep, these ideas need to be adjusted to one's personal characteristics. In addition, there are people whose duration of sleep can vary a lot, let's say from about 4-5 up to 8-9 hours. This last group of people may find it a little harder to apply these ideas related to voluntary sleep restriction. However, for most people, duration of sleep is consistent and corresponds to their breathing parameters as suggested by the table above.

After this theoretical consideration of the topic, here are practical examples that will guide you to activities required for implementation of these sleep-restriction methods.

Example A for a person with 15-20 s evening CP

Assume that a person, with about 15-20 s CP, usually goes to sleep at about 11 pm and wakes up at 7 am. How can he apply these sleep restriction ideas? Instead of going to sleep at 11 pm, he can practice another session of breathing exercises for 15-25 minutes at 11 pm. Or this person can practice informal reduced breathing and suitable breath holds (i.e., no need to record any numbers in the daily log), instead of going to sleep. What would be the expected reaction of the human body?

Normally, sleepiness, with yawning and desire to sleep, appears at about 11 pm and lasts for about 5-10 minutes. If he manages to stay awake and practice reduced breathing at this time, he should remain awake for the next hour. As a result, by 11:30 pm and midnight, he is likely to have even higher CPs than usual. This will help him tolerate shorter sleep better.

Then at about midnight, he will again experience an even stronger bout of sleepiness. At this time, he can go to sleep, while setting an alarm clock to 3 am. After waking up in the middle of the night, he needs to measure his CP and do a breathing session with mild or moderate air hunger for about 15-20 minutes. After the session, he can go to sleep setting the alarm clock at 6:30 am. With a 30 min break in sleep, the total duration for sleep in this example is 6 hours: 3 hours before the night break and 3 hours after.

Example B for a person with about 30 s evening CP

For someone with a higher CP (about 30 s), practical steps can be slightly different. Instead of doing a breathing session with a light or moderate air hunger, she may get most benefits from the breathing exercise that I call "Steps for adults" (see the book "Advanced Buteyko Breathing Exercises). Or she can do a breathing session that involve very long breath holds and strong air hunger. All these breathing exercises are described in the book "Advanced Buteyko Breathing Exercises". Otherwise, she can apply the same ideas related to staying awake for 1 hour and having this breathing session in the middle of the night after about 3 hours of sleep, with 6 hours of sleep in total.

Additional techniques to stay awake

There are, of course, many additional techniques to stay awake for 1 or 2 hours after your usual time when you go to sleep. Taking ice cold showers, even several times in row, is a great method to stay awake. This method is great to fall asleep fast, but keeping yourself more on the cold side can prevent or temporarily eliminate sleepiness.

Students worldwide drink a lot of coffee or very strong black tea to stay awake nearly all night in order to study before their exams. As a short-term technique, drinking coffee could be beneficial.

Another technique, that is more natural, is to play some light sport game or an active mental game or puzzle solving that will keep you awake for 1 or 2 hours. You need to be careful with all these methods since their overdose can keep you awake for too long time. This can later disrupt your circadian cycle, reduce your CP, and worsen your daily performance.

A good method to stay awake and increase CP is to go to some friendly dancing party. An atmosphere of mild excitement will help you avoid sleepiness. In addition, dancing with reduced breathing will help you to boost body CO_2 levels. Keep in mind though that you should not talk or do it very little to avoid CO_2 losses.

Barefoot walking, due to stimulation of nerve endings, can keep you awake for hours especially if you have not used this method during previous days or weeks. One or two minutes of barefoot walking can keep you awake for many hours later. Therefore, one needs to be careful in applying this method.

For people with poor blood sugar control and/or low weight

Generally, most people have no serious physiological or real problems with sleep restriction. They may have motivational problems or problems related to their will power. However, there are cases when these sleep-restriction methods can cause problems. For example, a person with low weight or poor blood sugar control can find that he cannot fall asleep after this middle-of-the-night breathing session. This happens due to a blood sugar drop after the session. Then falling asleep can be either very difficult or impossible.

The effect is likely to occur in those who have low body weight. In addition, there are those people who have nearly normal body weight, but due to not high enough CPs, their blood sugar control is not normal. Such people may also have periods of hypoglycemia with inability to fall asleep.

Such people may require a snack before or after the breathing session (done before sleep or in the middle of the night). Eating soft foods before breathing exercises or chewing food very well is a good solution. In this case, they can go to sleep immediately or shortly after the breathing session when the stomach gets empty.

If such a person does not have a snack before the breathing session, then he or she needs to have an after-the-session snack, and this snack should be digested before going to sleep. This is not an optimum solution since it causes a drop in one's CP. In such cases, using belts (or swaddling of adults) is a better choice to raise the morning CP.

5. Additional sleep factors

The methods and techniques from Chapter 4 are applied during sleep. However, there are many additional methods and factors that assist you to have better sleep and higher morning CP. This chapter describes these daytime techniques and factors. Note that nearly any activity that causes easier breathing and higher CP in the evening or before sleep is going to benefit quality of sleep and the morning CP. However, certain activities have an additional value due to their direct effect on a better quality of sleep.

5.1 Earlier supper

It is beneficial to have the last large daily meal earlier or up to 6-7 hours before you go to sleep. This allows you to achieve higher CPs before you go to sleep. In addition, you are going to spend more time just before sleep with higher CPs. If you get hungry later, let's say 1-2 hours before sleep, you can have a small snack that will be digested in about 30 minutes. Then you can again push your CP up with reduced breathing, pauses, and other breathing exercises.

Many people eat too late: at about 7 or 8 pm, they have a large supper. This is not a big problem if you apply the sleep restriction method described above in order to stay awake while trying to increase your CP to maximum numbers. However, since these people (who have large meals) go to sleep earlier, often at about 10-11 pm, their CP remains low for a long time due to digestion. After digestion, they have only a short period of time with higher CP.

This situation favors morning hyperventilation and needs to be avoided.

5.2 Reduced eating especially if you are overweight

In addition to having an earlier supper, you can have a smaller supper. This method helps to lose weight fast and is effective for people with extra weight.

You can eat about 2 times less than your usual meal and compensate or counteract your hunger (if any) by breathing exercises and higher CPs. As another option, you can reduce or eliminate fats and starches from your diet.

Reduced eating can also be applied during other parts of the day, not just before sleep. For example, if, on some days, your morning CP is too low, you can practice more breathwork before your breakfast to raise your blood sugar and energy levels naturally. When a person gets 30+ s CP, blood glucose control is much better, and blood glucose level is naturally at nearly normal levels. With 40+ s CP, weight loss can be very fast since it is much easier to exercise and there is nearly no hunger, especially for foods that are high in calories.

However, when the CP is less than 30 seconds, you need to be careful with this method. Many people found that if they do not eat enough and have slightly low blood glucose levels, they have much poorer sleep and may not fall asleep for up to 30-60 minutes. This can happen due to deliberate reduced eating before sleep, or during fasting, or during days of reduced eating.

5.3 Physical exercise for shorter and better sleep

As it is discussed on web pages of NormalBreathing.com devoted to physical exercise, at over 20 s CP, correct physical exercise becomes the key factor for further progress. Physical activity becomes even more important than breathing exercises. These pages also provide details and tables related to the link between physical exercise and breathing patterns. In particular, prolonged physical exercise has a powerful effect on the next morning CP. Therefore, it is a very important factor for shorter and better sleep.

Are there any additional ideas related to positive effects of physical exercise on better and shorter sleep? It is beyond the scope of this book to describe all these effects, yet certain crucial factors need to be mentioned.

First of all, exhausting physical activity, such as over 2 hours of strenuous continuous running or some other very intensive type of exercise may require long recovery and are often not optimum forms of exercise even when all exercise is done with nose breathing. (These negative effects can be eliminated if one uses the Training Mask - see the related web page for more details: http://www.normalbreathing.com/d/training-mask.php).

However, without the use of the Training Mask, it is healthier to have a slightly reduced intensity of exercise, and to do it with, apart from nose breathing, additional breath control or breathing less. Also, it is better to spread exercise over 2-3 or even 4 sessions.

Second, some forms of exercise, such as games, can cause problems with sleep if they over-activate the sympathetic nervous system and are done within a few hours before sleep. For example, if you did not play basketball or other games for some weeks, an active game for 1 hour somewhere around 7-8 pm or later can make you over-excited and keep you agitated for several hours later. Mild over-stimulation can be a positive factor for sleep restriction, as we mentioned above. But excessive agitation can prevent you from sleeping for many hours.

5.4 Diet, nutrition and supplements

Diet and nutrition and their effects on breathing and health, are other large topics that you can study using other sources. A balanced raw vegetarian (or even better, vegan) diet is a positive factor that allows better and shorter sleep naturally. This is a general factor that helps to get higher morning CPs.

For people with low CPs (less than 20 s), supplementation with all missing or required nutrients will definitely improve their sleep. Certain nutrients, such as fish oil (or its components, EPA and DHA) can directly influence the next morning CP. Many breathing students discovered that a tablespoon of fish oil per day, after 3-5 days, can increase their morning CPs by 3-7 s, in some cases, up to 10 seconds.

Therefore, it is important to find out more about signs and symptoms of various common deficiencies. It is also useful to learn how to apply the 3-day test in order to test yourself in relation to prevalent deficiencies, such as deficiencies in magnesium, calcium, zinc and fish oil.

Low levels of blood cortisol have a negative effect of quality of sleep causing a large CP drop. This effect takes place in predisposed people or those who have severe or prolonged problems with inflammation, stress and/or adrenal fatigue. The criteria and exact techniques related to finding the initial cortisol dosage, supplementation regime, and safe weaning-off cortisol at higher CPs can be found in other sources.

5.5 Cold shower before sleep and during the day

It is known that there are a lot of people who do not tolerate cold conditions. They easily catch respiratory infections. These are often those people who have nearly no **brown fat cells** left in their bodies due to the prolonged absence of cold stimulation. This group of people often uses warm or too warm blankets causing overheating and overbreathing during sleep.

Brown fat cells have a very high concentration of mitochondria. As a result, these cells are able to generate heat at rest. This ability is especially important during cold weather conditions and sleep in cold conditions.

Brown fat is an area of very active research with 100s of teams of scientists trying to find ways to increase brown fat content in the human body since brown fat helps to deal with heart disease, obesity, diabetes and many other problems.

You can get increased numbers of brown fat cells naturally by taking regular cold showers. Note that this process is very gradual. Eventually, you can adapt to sleeping in cold conditions comfortably.

Taking a cold shower before sleep will help you to sleep in colder conditions and have a higher morning CP. Cold showers can be also used in order to apply the sleep restriction methods, as it was described above. Remember the crucial safety rules related to taking a cold shower:
- normal blood sugar levels
- good wellbeing and over 20 seconds for your current CP
- warming up bones, first, if they are cold when you go to the shower
- gradual application of cold water so that to have a smooth extended transition to cooling.

For explanation and other details related to safe use of a cold shower, visit the web page that explains correct and safe application of cold showers.

5.6 Walk in fresh air

For many people, especially those who spent limited time outdoors (e.g., only 1-2 hours), having a walk or easy physical exercise outdoors before sleep (preferably within 1 hour before sleep) is an additional assisting factor that helps them to fall asleep faster and improve sleep quality.

About 10-12 minutes spent outdoors are enough to produce beneficial effects, but many people get maximum benefits if the spend up to 20-30 minutes in the fresh air.

6. Examples of sleep positions and swaddling

First let us consider practical examples of various sleep positions.

6.1 Horizontal sleep postures

There are usually not many problems with horizontal sleep positions. Ideally, we try to alternate between the left side and the chest.

There is, however, an intermediate position that is called "Falcon". This horizontal sleep position is shown below.

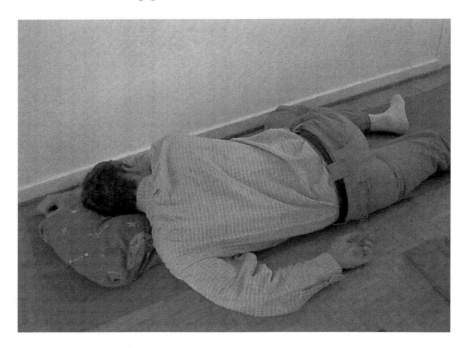

As you can see, this is a partially left side position: the left side of the chest takes the highest pressure from to the body trunk.

As a result, one can also have the same position on the right side of the chest. Furthermore, it is possible to alternate between these 2 positions during sleep.

The right "Falcon" sleep posture is as good as prone (chest) or left side sleep.

6.2 Sitting sleep positions

The situation with sitting postures is more complicated. First of all, let us look at examples of chairs that can be used for sleep.

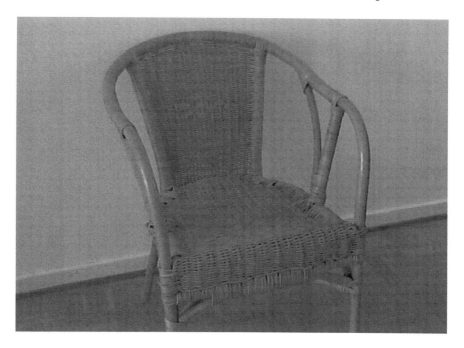

The chair above is not suitable for following reasons. First, there is very little support for the elbows and lower arms.

Second, the chair is sagging. This means that it will prevent sliding down due to the elevation of the front part of the chair. This frontal part of this chair will greatly reduce blood flow into the legs.

However, if you are very motivated, tired (due to a lot of daily exercise), and sleepy, you can probably "survive" on this chair through the whole night.

The next image shows the application of this chair for sleep.

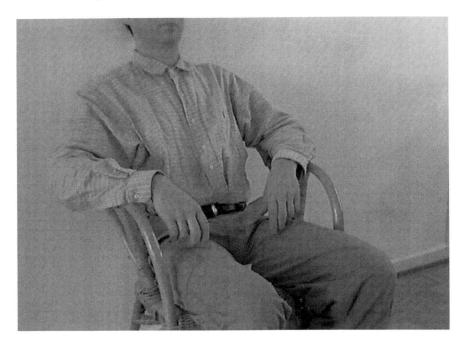

For the above image, **the head is propped against the wall**. That is not so bad, but quite unstable: the head can drop to the left or right side and become unsupported.

The arms are only partially supported by the chair.

The middle parts of both thighs are under pressure due to the front edge of the chair. This can cause problems with circulation during prolonged sleep.

It is possible to solve this problem of reduced circulation for this chair by stretching legs as shown below.

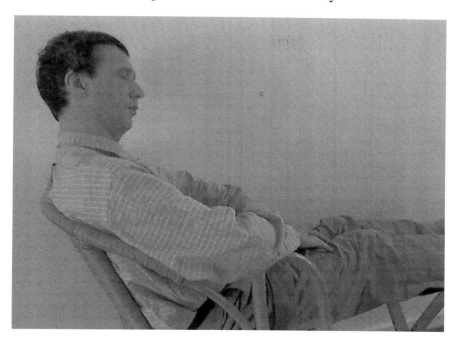

Large disadvantages of this sleep position are: the unsupported head and poorly supported arms (too high pressure on a small areas of both arms). The frontal part of this chair still presses hard against the legs causing reduced blood flow.

This is a better chair for sleeping (below).

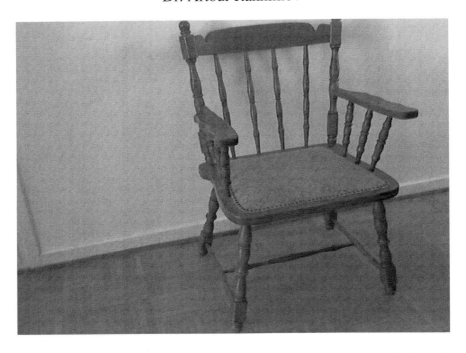

It has a better support for the elbows and lower arms. In addition, the seat of this chair is flat.

Here is the picture showing how to use this chair for sleep.

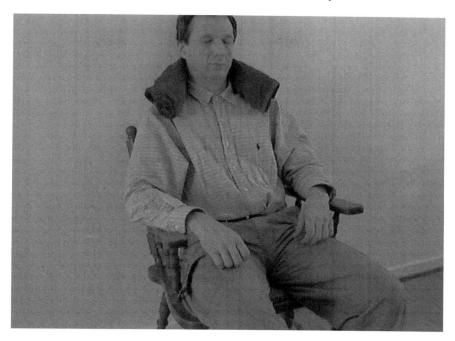

You may notice that this chair allows more relaxation. The head is resting against the wall and is, in addition, supported by the towel. This towel can be inserted in a pillow case. Alternatively, one may use a semi-circular pillow.

(Make sure that any fabric that is in contact with your skin is cotton or some other natural fabric.)

For the above chair, the arms get much better support in comparison with the previous chair.

The flat seat allows better relaxation of the legs.

Here is another example with the same chair.

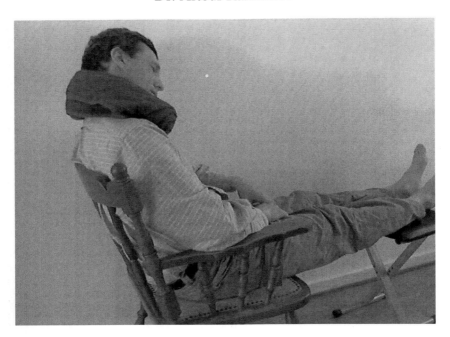

While there is no wall support for the head, the pillow takes most of the pressure from the head. The legs are stretched forward. (Note that keeping the legs down makes the posture closer to standing and is better for breathing and higher body O2. Therefore, if possible, avoid stretching legs forward.)

Many couches and sofas can also be used for sleeping sitting. Here is an example.

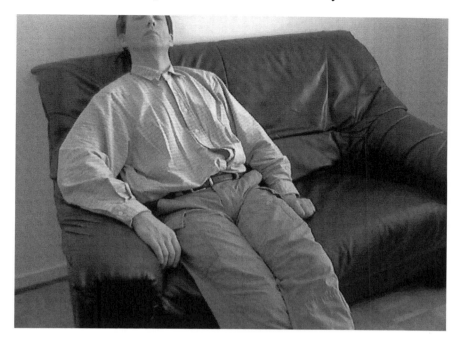

As we can see here, the head has some partial support.

The right arm is propped by the side of the sofa. However, the left arm is poorly supported. Only its lower parts are propped by the surface of the sofa.

This position will still likely keep your CP high.

However, if you use a chair or something else to support your stretched forward legs, then your sleep posture will be similar to a reclining position with a nearly 45 degree angle. This position is very unlikely to prevent overbreathing.

Therefore, while the above position looks like an inclined one, it still works well to keep one's CP high.

You can find more information about sleep positions in Chapter 7: Questions and Answers.

Now we can turn our attention to swaddling. As we discussed above, the purpose of swaddling (for adults too) is to prevent overbreathing and/or chest breathing during sleep. The degree and rigorousness of this technique depends mainly on the current CP, usual CP drop at night, and the desired goals. Let me provide examples so you can more easily understand the main principles and ideas behind effects of swaddling.

6.3 Swaddling for people with very low morning CPs

Adults with about 15 s CP breathe nearly 15 L/min at rest, while sitting. After transition into a horizontal position, during the initial period of sleep, due to reduced metabolism, their minute ventilation slightly decreases. The CP remains about the same.

However, with increased duration of sleep, after some hours of sleep, the CP starts to decrease. This happens due to heavier or increased breathing. One can easily observe and hear heavy breathing of sick people during sleep.

With less than 10 s CP, it is common to have a minute ventilation of over 20 liters per minute at rest and during sleep too. For many severely sick people, any horizontal position makes their breathing heavier. This is one of the key reasons why these critically ill people are most likely to have acute exacerbations and can even die during sleep.

For all these groups of people with less than 15 s for their usual daily CPs, their breathing during sleep becomes so heavy that even a single belt located on the lower ribs is able to prevent severe overbreathing and reduce the CP drop.

Let us consider a practical example.

A person with an inflammatory condition and about 15 s evening CP has only about 5-6 s for his morning CP. To prevent this large overnight CP drop, he started to tape his mouth and apply the technique to prevent supine sleep at night. These methods increased

108

his morning CP to 8-9 seconds. He noticed fewer symptoms and reduction in their intensity. In order to further improve his morning CP, he decided to apply one belt during sleep.

After applying this swaddling technique with one belt, this person found that his morning CP increased from about 8-9 seconds up to 12 seconds. This image shows the position of the belt (on the middle of his body trunk) for the whole duration of his sleep (about 8 hours).

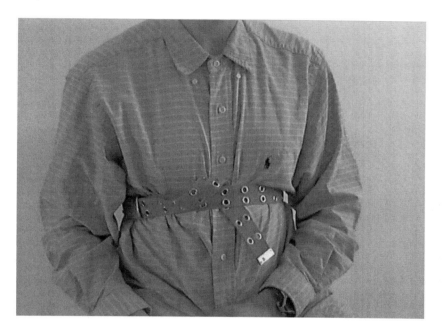

Note that one belt did not completely prevent his overnight CP drop, but it reduced this drop about 2 times. Indeed, without a belt, his CP decreased: from 15 s to 8-9 s. With this simple one-belt method, his morning CP increased from about 8-9s to 12 seconds.

Since the same positive effect can be achieved on the following nights as well, the overall or accumulative effect of one belt, after 1-2 weeks, can be large. Obviously, an improvement in the morning CP after weeks or months of training is the key factor that measures and reflects one's health progress.

For example, without using a belt, this man would normally get about 2-3 seconds weekly increase for his morning CP. After application of the belt, he got a 7-10 second improvement in his morning CP. In other words, his overall progress became 2-3 times greater. This is a significant health booster especially if we take into account that this method does not require a lot of additional time.

However, when this man got to about 20 s for his morning CP, a single belt did not provide any significant further improvements. Sleeping with a single belt or without it produced about the same morning CPs.

What could be the reason? With 20 s for his morning CP, this man started to breathe, during the early morning hours, about 2 times less air than 1-2 weeks ago when his morning CP was 10 s.

Therefore, when the morning CP gets higher (e.g., about 20 seconds), we need to use more rigorous or more restrictive methods for prevention of overbreathing at night.

6.4 Using 2 or more belts for swaddling during sleep

Of course, one can use 2 or 3 belts with lower CPs as well. This will produce even better results in comparison with the case described in the previous section of this book.

When using 2 or more belts, the position of the main belt is the same: it is located on the middle of the trunk or just above 3 lower ribs (at the level of the spleen and liver). The position of other belts depends on the effects of the main belt.

When a person uses one tight belt in the middle of the trunk, he or she cannot take a large or deep breath using the lower rib cage. As a result, most people start to use their abdominal and diaphragmatic breathing muscles. However, some people, especially elderly women, start to breathe using their upper chest. Therefore, we need to apply two different strategies that depend on this transformation related to a new breathing pattern.

A. For most people (who become abdominal breathers)

These people do not have problems with upper chest breathing. Hence, they should use additional belts below the main belt (between lower ribs and the belly button or navel).

Here is an image that shows one additional (black) belt located below the main. As you can see, the additional belt is located between the main belt and the belly button.

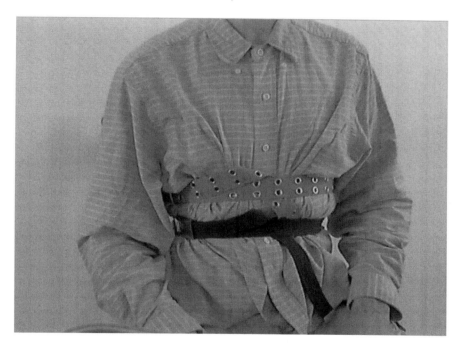

It is also possible and more effective to use additional belts. For example, this image shows a third (blue) belt. This blue belt is added just above the belly button.

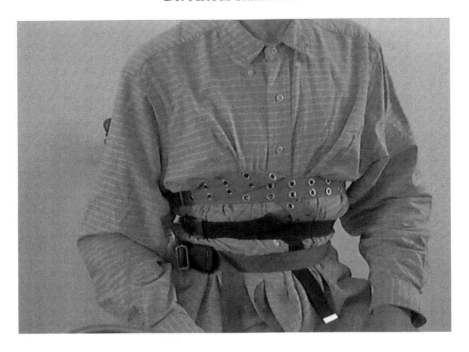

More belts further restrict breathing during sleep reducing or even preventing the overnight CP drop.

Many people are fine with belts and use them for many days in a row without any problems. However, some people discover that they need to make belts too tight to keep their CPs high. As a result, these people cannot endure their tight belts during the whole night. If this is a case with you, then it is also possible to use a swaddling vest that uniformly distributes extra pressure and is much easier to tolerate for several hours of sleep. You can find details about making a swaddling vest below.

B. For those who are upper chest breathers

If you discovered that an application of one belt makes you an upper chest breather, you need to apply a second belt above the main belt or under your armpits in order to prevent upper chest breathing. The purpose of the belts in this case is to ensure abdominal breathing during sleep.

Here is an image that demonstrates 2 belts: the main belt (for lower ribs) and another one located under armpits and on the upper chest.

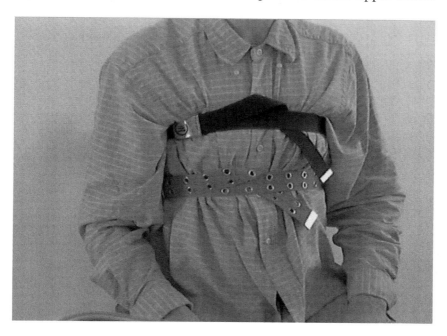

For people with less than 30 s for the morning CP, it is very common to breathe using their chests at night. In such cases, they can use 3 belts located on the rib cage. For men, these 3 belts can be between the nipples and the lowest rib. For women, 2 belts can be under the breasts and one above the breasts, with additional belts (if necessary) under armpits.

It is also clear that abdominal breathing needs to be adopted by the body. It is actually a serious shift in your breathing mechanics and the operation of many organs located under the diaphragm.

After 1 week of sleep with these 2 belts that "force" abdominal breathing, you will likely not need the belt under the armpits. Following one week of "training" (using these 2 belts), you can start to gradually restrict your abdominal breathing without the danger of upper chest breathing. But keep in mind that your transition should

113

be gradual. If you are worried about upper chest breathing at night, you can apply the armpit belt as well as abdominal belts.

6.5 Degree of swaddling and morning CP

Sometimes, very motivated breathing students are able to improve their morning CPs due to very rigorous application of belts or other swaddling methods during sleep (other techniques are provided below). If you notice that after swaddling it is hard to take your usual breath, then it is possible that your breathing will become lighter after being swaddled for many hours or during sleep.

However, for most people, the degree of physical discomfort, due to pressure from belts or other devices, makes falling asleep and sleeping difficult. As a result, the optimum solution is to find those conditions for swaddling that are on the limits of your tolerance or comfort.

As we can see the effects are following. You can use less pressure and fewer belts, but then your morning-CP results will have only light or unacceprably moderate improvements. Or you can apply a lot of pressure with many belts (or while using other methods described below) with great CP results, but with some physical and mental discomfort.

6.6 Criteria and area for swaddling

What is the exact criteria that makes swaddling effective? Good swaddling is characterized by 2 requirements:

1. You notice that you cannot take a deep or bigger breath after swaddling is applied.

2. It is difficult to insert a finger between a belt (or other device) and your T-shirt or sleeping shirt. In other words, if you try to insert a finger between a belt and your shirt, you need to apply considerable pressure to achieve that.

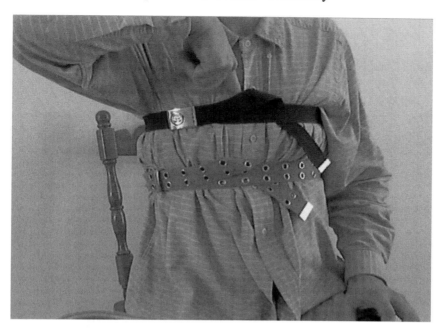

The area of restriction is from the navel to nipples in men, and from the navel to breasts in women. The total time should not exceed 8-10 hours per day. Thus, the restriction can be done during nights or some parts of days. Day-time restriction can be a useful reminder for severely sick patients with poor memory or with stressful work (Souliagin, 1991a).

Warning: People with **inflammatory bowel disease (Crohn's disease and ulcerative colitis**), duodenal ulcers, and some other digestive conditions should not apply pressure on their belly and digestive organs if this pressure causes a flare-up and/or worsening of their symptoms. This is particularly dangerous during active exacerbations of the gut (flare-ups) characterized by inflammation, abnormal peristalsis and shortened transition time with diarrhea. In these and other similar situations with active existing damage to internal organs, only the ribs are the safe areas for mechanical restriction of ventilation. However, after or during partial recovery, this group of people can tolerate mild or even strong pressure on their abdominal areas without negative effects.

6.7 Type of belts for swaddling

There are many types of belts and straps that can be used for swaddling. Keep in mind that we can use only **unstretchable belts** in order to prevent problems with circulation and only for a certain period of time.

Here is a short review of these gadgets so that it is easier for student to choose the right belts.

Ordinary belts

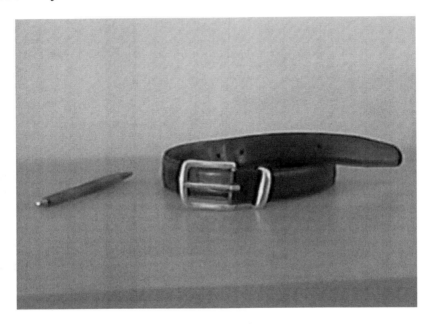

These types of belts are not suitable for overnight swaddling. You can use ordinary belts during the daytime (to remind yourself about abdominal breathing) or during breathing exercises (when practicing Buteyko exercises, or with the Frolov and other breathing devices). If you try to use such a belt at night, the belt may last just for a few nights, after which, the hole(s) will be too large due to mechanical damage.

Fortified belts with metal holes

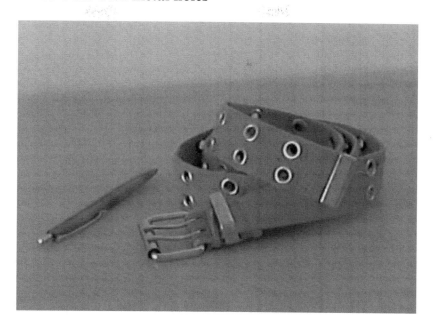

There are many varieties of such belts. They can be called "Army Green Metal Buckle Double 2-Rows Belt Strap", "Brown Punk Two Rows Metal Holes Belt", "Brown Leather Biker Belt with 2 Rows of BIG Metal Eyelets" and so forth.

These are belts suitable for overnight swaddling. They can last for some weeks or even months depending on the strength of these belts and the pressure that is applied. Another disadvantage of these belts is that the holes are about 2-3 cm apart. This means that they may not be exactly what you need. In addition, if you want to have good swaddling, it is not easy to lock these belts. You may need a complete exhalation to make these belts tight.

Buckle straps

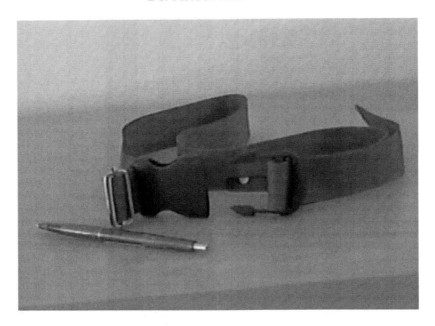

Buckle straps can also do a great job. Some of them may not be able to withstand a high pressure: they can become unlocked during an inhalation or when changing a position during sleep. Thus, you need to select those buckle straps that can withstand higher pressure.

Alligator Belt Straps

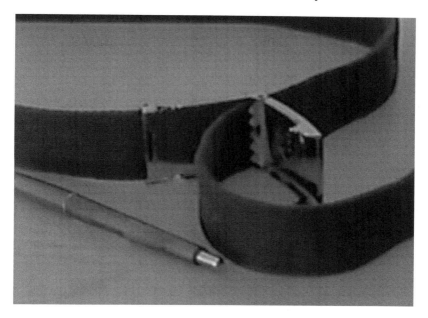

These are usually called "Alligator Belt Straps" or "Alligator Straps". These are probably the most suitable belts or straps for swaddling since they are strong, durable, adjustable to any length, and flat (do not create too much pressure and stress for the body trunk).

Pressure from belts

For most belts, one of the problems relate to the large size of the buckle part. During sleep, this hard part of the belt will produce much higher pressure on the body trunk. The natural tendency is to leave all these buckles and solid parts of the bed on your chest. Then it is uncomfortable to sleep on the chest, especially if you sleep on a hard surface.

To solve this challenge, you can move these hard parts of the belts to the right side, as it is shown in the image.

119

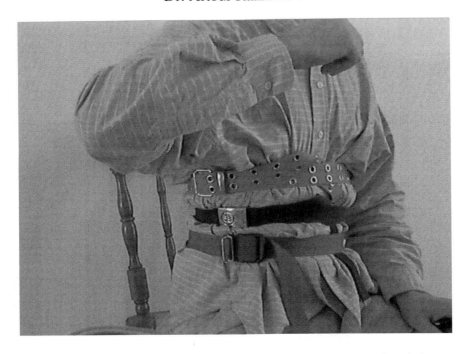

This positioning of belts often helps prevent sleeping on the right side, which is not as good as the left side (unless you have your heart located on the right side). The method will work better if you sleep on a really hard surface.

While using belts is the most common method of swaddling, there are other techniques that sometimes can be more effective than belts. Let us consider two additional methods.

6.8 How to make a swaddling vest

One of the methods is based on the use of a strong shirt or T-shirt that is made of denim fabric. Note that some varieties of denim fabric are too thin. For swaddling, you need to find the thick types of denim that can withstand high tearing or stretching pressure.

Here is a possible example of a starting vest that you need to modify:

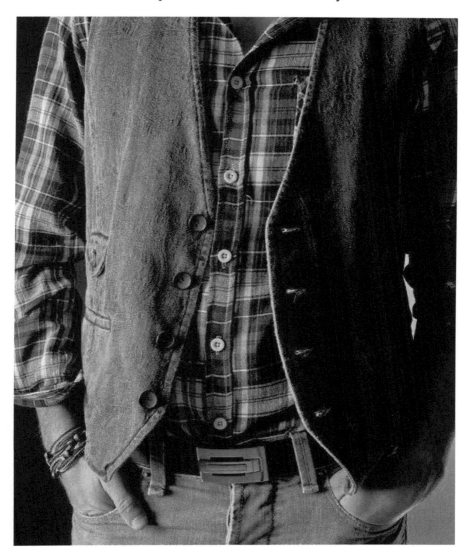

You can choose such a shirt or vest so that, if you can close all 4 buttons, this creates light pressure on your body trunk. In other words, you need a shirt or vest that is tight for you to wear. Of course, a normal shirt (for wearing) will be a little bit loose (but without any noticeable pressure on the body trunk).

You can even select a very tight vest or shirt that is of a smaller size.

For good swaddling, we need to make additional steps so that this vest can prevent overbreathing during sleep. In order for this vest to work, we need much higher pressure when the buttons are closed (so that you can not take a deeper breath using chest at all and/or even your usual abdominal breathing feels restricted). We also need a stronger connection between the buttons and the denim fabric. Ordinary buttons will not keep high pressure for a long time because their threads or attachment methods are not strong enough.

Here is a step-by-step guide.

1. Find or buy a denim vest that is very tight for you. It can be something like what you see below.

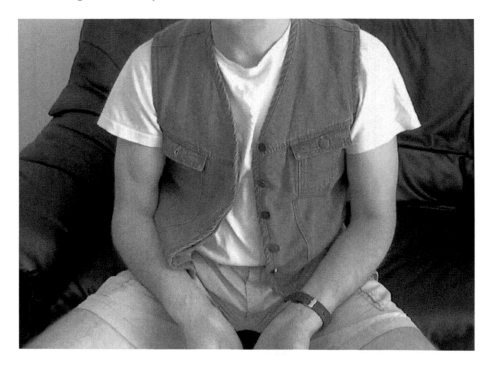

Even though this is a small denim vest, it is necessary to add buttons to make it tight for the lower body trunk.

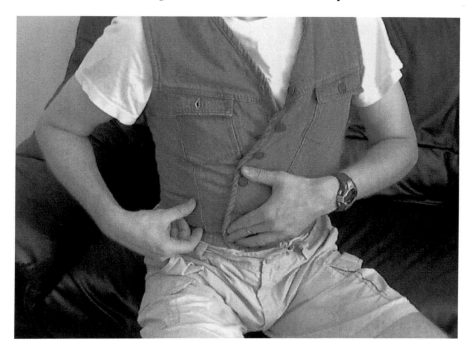

The image above demonstrated the width of a piece of material (with buttons) that can be cut out from this vest.

The next image shows how much extra material can be removed.

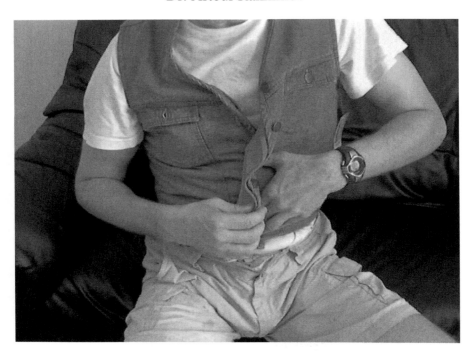

When this material is removed, you will get an even smaller vest, as the next image demonstrates.

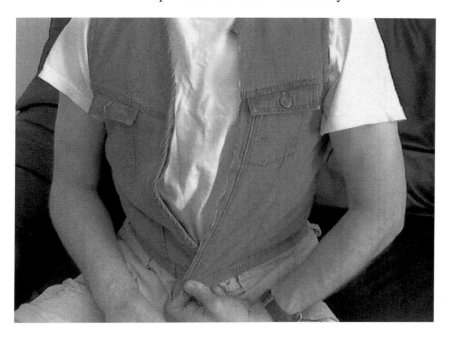

Now the buttons are removed (see above), and you may notice a fresh cut on the left part of the vest. (It is on the right side on the above image.)

The next step is to find **the right positions for new buttons** which will be used for swaddling. You need to try to make the lowest part of the vest as tight as possible in order to find out the places for new buttons. The buttons from the left and right side should be about 5 cm (2 inches) apart.

After the sides of the vest are brought together (see the image below), the thumbs show approximate positions for the lowest buttons.

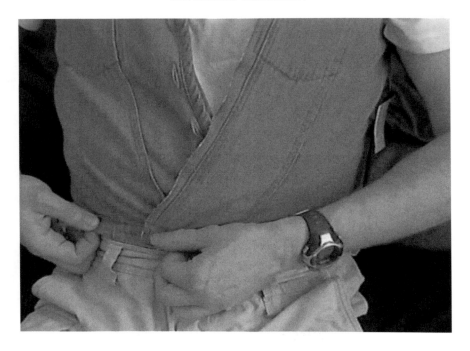

The left-side buttons will be sewn along the left edge of the vest.

Here is the result:

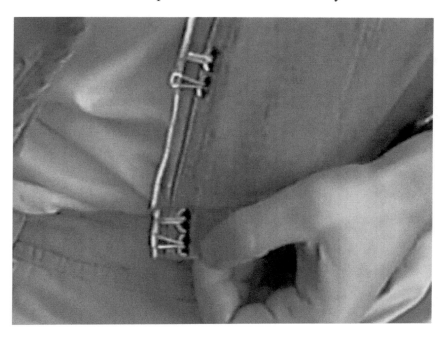

The right buttons should be at least 5 cm away from the left buttons when the vest is tight (as on the above image). Then there is a gap to connect the left and right buttons with a rope to make the vest tight.

The next image shows the 2 added lower right buttons. When I simply attach the left side (without too much pressure), there is a large gap between left and right buttons.

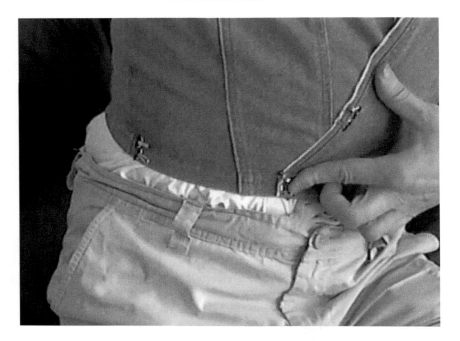

For this specific vest, the intended design is to have 3 pairs of buttons on the left side and 3 pairs on the right side.

Here is what was created.

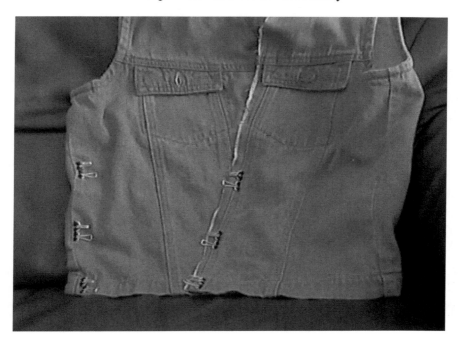

The vest in use

When you put this vest on connect the buttons using a rope. Which kind of rope should one choose? **Shoe laces** work fine for this job. Why is this so? Shoe laces are very strong. They can be adjusted to any desired length (but not too long, of course). They are designed to be tied and stay in the same position under long cyclic pressure.

The next image shows the same vest tied with 3 shoe laces.

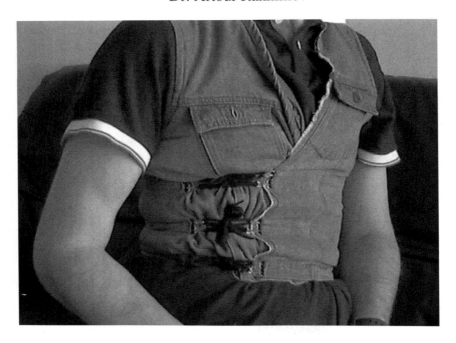

From this last image, we can also get ideas for the type of buttons to use. For this vest, hook-and-eye buttons are used. But they were not sewn in order to be connected with each other. As you may notice, for each pair of neighboring buttons (located next to each other), the lower button is an eye button, while the upper button is a hook button.

This was done with a purpose. In order to close this vest, you need to tie all three sets of buttons using laces.

The above image also shows the main weakness of this vest. You may notice that the right side of the body trunk is under strong pressure created by the right-side buttons. This is because the body trunk has an uneven curvature. The frontal part and the back are nearly flat, and these body parts do not get high pressure even if you make a very tight swaddling. The main pressure goes to both sides. For the above image, the left-side buttons are located near the middle line for the frontal part of the body. Therefore, the left side of the body trunk gets more homogeneous pressure distribution.

The right side has buttons that are at the place of the largest curvature. Therefore, these right buttons create high pressure and may cause discomfort during sleep (depending on motivation, tightness of swaddling and other factors).

How to close this vest with laces

First, insert the lace into the lower eye-buttons at the top of the vest and tighten them as shown in the image below.

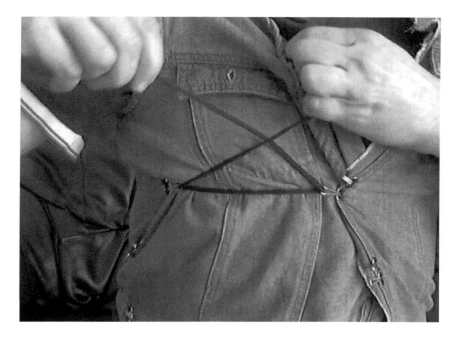

Then the lower eye buttons are tightened. You need to put the lace through hooks (or 2 upper buttons) and tighten the lace again.

The next step is to tie the upper lace (see the image below).

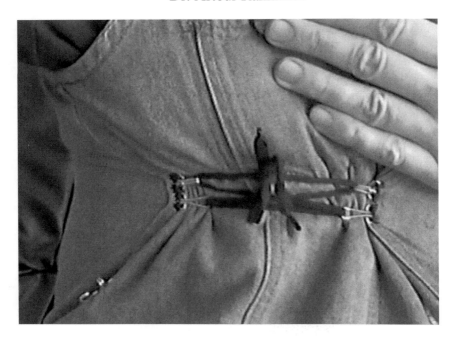

Then you need to repeat the same process for the buttons located in the middle area of the vest.

Finally, you need to tie the lower buttons.

If you want to make a vest that has more homogeneous pressure distribution, you can make 4, 5, 6 or even 7 sets of buttons.

If you wish to make the vest even tighter, you can repeat the process from the top and the bottom. In fact, when there are 3-4 or more sets of buttons, you can notice that after you tied all buttons, the tops ones become slightly loose. This is because pressure from the lower buttons constricts the rib cage. Therefore, you may repeat the process starting from the top and achieve really good swaddling.

Where and how to sew buttons to make a tough vest

Since the vest should withstand high pressure for many nights (up to months), then we require:

1) a strong or very strong thread for sewing the buttons

2) a place that has at least double, triple, or quadruple layers so that the pressure from the buttons is homogeneously distributed over a larger area of denim fabric.

Which other buttons can be used?

Hook-and-eye buttons are a good choice because they are attached to a large area of denim fabric. Of course, it is sensible to find either **large or medium size hook-and-eye buttons** to make a swaddling vest. In this particular design, **No. 9 Hook-and-Eye Buttons** were used. Small buttons may not be suitable for our purposes.

However, if you cannot easily find the correct hook-and-eye buttons, you can also use large and strong ordinary **round buttons** preferably with 4 or more holes.

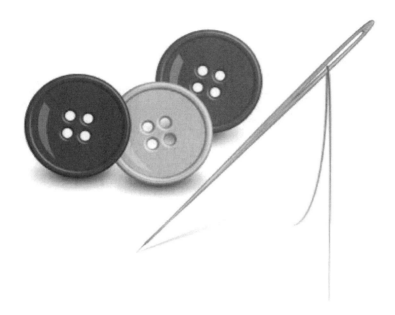

6.9 Best swaddling vest (a new method)

Some people are able to use 2-3 belts and consistently get great CP improvements with these belts. However, belts create high pressure on the sides of the body.

Many breathing students, due to their strong motivation, are ok with this pressure. However, many other students can wear belts only for some 2-4 hours of sleep. Later during the night, these students wake up and cannot fall asleep due to pressure and discomfort created by the belts. These 2-4 hours of swaddling still provide health benefits, but there are better solutions in order to remain swaddled for the whole duration of sleep.

When the swaddling vest is done with buttons, as we discussed above, this pressure is distributed over a larger area of the body trunk. However, there are still considerable pressure variations that are felt on the sides of the body. In order to solve this challenge, one can add many more sets of buttons in order to make pressure more homogeneous.

An even better solution is to use, instead of belts or buttons, something that uniformly holds two opposite sides of the vest together. How can we achieve this?

You can attach the opposite sides of the swaddling vest with **velcro fabric straps**. Here is a picture of a ready-to-use vest.

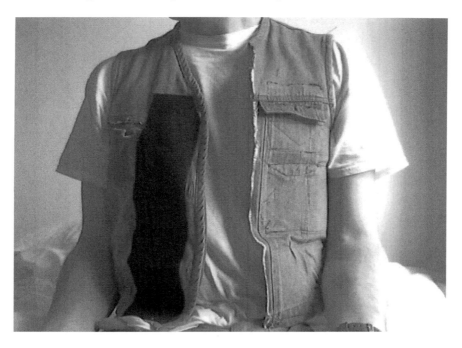

The vest is made of blue denim fabric. On the right side of this vest (the left side on the image above), you can see a large strip of black velcro.

The supplementary layer of velcro is hidden on the inner surface of the opposite side.

Here is an image below that shows the inner hidden velcro layers. These 4 velcro straps are also black and you can easily see them.

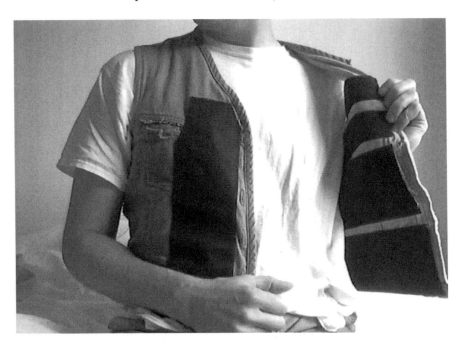

When applied and closed, this vest creates very homogeneous pressure.

Here is an image of the closed vest.

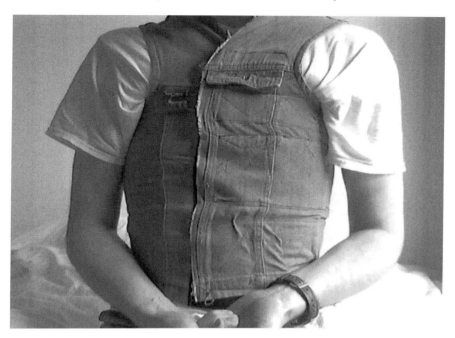

It is important to make a **forceful (nearly maximum) exhalation** before joining velcro strips of the opposite side of this vest. Then this vest will be tight, and it will prevent rib cage expansions during inhalations.

Of course, one needs to use a strong thread and sew velcro straps 2-3 times along the perimeter. In addition, each strap can be sewn in their middle parts, in a zigzag or some other pattern, so as to improve connection between the velcro fabric and the denim fabric.

Dimensions of straps

The purpose of the vest is to prevent expansion of the rib cage during inhalations while sleeping. Therefore, the attached area of contact between opposite velcro straps should be at least 2-3 cm wide (about 1 inch). This is possible and easy if you choose right velcro straps that are wide enough, and attach these velcro straps in right positions.

137

For the velcro vest described in this book, the following dimensions were used:
- the right-side strap (the left side in the image) is 10 cm (4 inches) wide and 36 cm long (nearly 12 inches). Here is its image again.

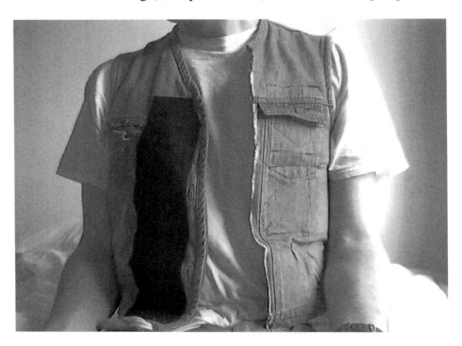

By using a wider strap, it is easier to adjust pressure from very low to moderate and high.

The inner left side of the vest has 4 velcro straps attached to it: 2 wide ones below, and 2 narrower ones above.

The lower (larger) straps are about 10 by 21 cm in size (or 4 by 8.5 inches). The top 2 straps are 5 cm wide (2 inches). They are 19 and 11 cm long. The smallest velcro strap is at the top.

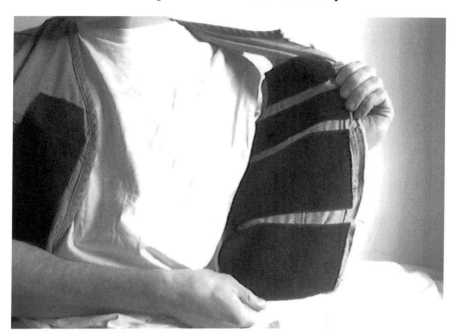

These 4 straps on the left side have gaps between them. These gaps allow us to move the straps making the vest tighter or less tight depending on our intentions.

Among all suggested designs (using belts, buttons and velcro), this last design is the most comfortable one. It is much easier to tolerate such vests for the whole duration of sleep even when they create high pressure.

6.10 Possible problems due to swaddling

The majority of breathing students do not have significant problems with correctly applied swaddling. They wake up in the morning while still being swaddled feeling that their breath is light and their morning CP is high.

However, some students may find swaddling difficult and uncomfortable. They may remove their belts during the night. These incidents usually have physiological causes.

139

Let us consider some of these **negative physiological or environmental factors**.

- **Too warm sleeping conditions**. If your blanket is too warm, then your respiratory rate and minute ventilation will gradually increase during sleep. If you wake up some hours later noticing that swaddling becomes too restrictive, check your CP and your sensation of warmness. If your CP dropped and you feel warm, you are likely overheated. As a result of overheating causing heavy breathing, swaddling creates too much pressure and discomfort. This breathing student may blame swaddling for the problem and not use it anymore. However, in reality, the solution is to have cooler conditions for sleep. To prevent overheating, use cooler clothes and blankets during sleep. Remember that, with over 20 s CP, it is important and healthy to sleep in colder conditions.

- **Carpets in your bedroom**. Presence of carpets makes air quality tens or even hundreds of times worse. During a night's sleep several cubic meters of air with millions or billions of **airborne particles, including dust, dust mites, their droppings, bacteria, viruses, etc**. will enter through the nasal passages making them dryer. These airborne particles penetrate into bronchi and the lungs causing stress for the immune system and leading to deeper breathing. Most people have good tolerance to these adverse factors. In other words, they do not experience strong reactions to dust, dust mites, mold and other airborne particles. However, other people experience allergic reactions, which make breathing heavier. Sleeping in carpet-free rooms or covering carpets with plastic will solve this problem. You can also wear a thick dust mask during sleep. It can make your inhaled air much cleaner.

- **Very dusty pillow cases, blankets, and bed sheets** create the same effect, as do **books, newspapers, hanging clothes, and old dusty curtains**. Make sure that your bedroom has good air quality.

- **Closed windows during the night** greatly worsen air quality in the bedroom due to poor air circulation and absence of air ions that make air cleaner. Either keep windows open or, if it is too cold or too noisy outside, buy an air ionizer/purifier and keep it running throughout the night.

If you are able to fall asleep and sleep for 1-2 hours, but wake up later feeling that swaddling is too difficult to tolerate, then there is some other cause that relates to intensification of your breathing during sleep. Many common causes of this overbreathing are considered above. However, there are some other factors that can make your breathing deeper. If you encounter this challenge, you may need to analyze and think about other possible causes of your night overbreathing.

6.9 Three major factors that make swaddling easier to tolerate

There are 3 major **positive factors that makes swaddling easier to tolerate**.

- **Higher evening CP:** If you have higher evening CP numbers (due to intensive breathing exercises before sleep), then your breathing will be lighter. As a result, even very rigorous swaddling will be easier to tolerate. Therefore, practice more sessions before sleep for easier breathing during sleep and do dozens of other things that increase your evening CP.

- **More physical exercise during the day:** If you do more exercise with nose breathing (even better with the Training Mask: http://www.normalbreathing.com/d/training-mask.php), then your breathing will be lighter during sleep assisting easier forbearance of swaddling. As it was described earlier, more physical exercise usually does not cause an immediate increase in one's CP. The effects of intensive or prolonged exercise are reflected on one's next morning CP (unless one uses the Training Mask). This is exactly the factor that allows longer sleep (up to 5-7 hours) without a large increase in minute ventilation.

- **Electrical grounding (Earthing) during sleep**: Most people are going to get benefits and have easier breathing with better body oxygenation and better tolerance in relation to swaddling if they use Earthing.

Apart from these physiological factors, one's motivation is also an important assisting factor. If you imagine all the health benefits of a high CP when going to sleep, you can increase your tolerance threshold.

6.10 Crucial rules related to swaddling

1. If you have even slight anxiety or uneasiness about the swaddling method, **start your swaddling program gradually**. Get lightly swaddled about 20-40 min before sleep and practice relaxation of the diaphragm (abdominal muscles) or reduced breathing until you go to sleep. It is important that your mind and body are relaxed and positive in relation to swaddling. On the following days, you can increase pressure so that you feel that your breathing is more and more restricted.

2. Use swaddling either during the day or during the night for up to **no more than a total of 8 hours per day**. You can wear a belt with very low pressure at other times just to remind you about breathing less and about abdominal breathing.

3. You can **use swaddling for up to 2-3 weeks**, but then you need to take a break that should be of about the same duration (2-3 weeks).

4. Use swaddling **when you try to increase your morning CP**, but not as a long term strategy to maintain your morning CP. This means that once you achieve a higher morning CP, you need to switch to natural methods and techniques (not swaddling, but, for example, exercise and cold shower) that allow you to preserve this CP later. With higher morning CPs, it is easier to do more physical exercise and practice informal reduced breathing (i.e., outside your formal breathing sessions). These are most influential factors that will help you to maintain higher morning CPs later.

Common examples of situations when swaddling is smart to use are:
- in order to quickly recover from an infection that causes overbreathing and a large drop in a morning CP
- in order to recover from an exposure to allergies, a trip to some place (with a CP drop), a period of unhealthy eating, etc.
- during cleansing reactions (as discussed above)
- when advancing to higher CP zones (trying to get 20+ s for the morning CP, 30+, and 50+).

7. Questions and answers about sleep, symptoms, and breathing

Here are some questions posted on the NormalBreathing site in the past with expanded answers here.

7.1 Sleep stages and duration of sleep

Q: You write that persons with a high CP don't remember dreams and have no nightmares. In the last few weeks I got my CP from 10 to 17 s. After getting from 15 to 17 I suddenly started to have very alive dreaming. I remember a lot of my dreams and I kind of like that. Before I almost did not dream or only remembered the last few minutes. I guess I am an exception here. I wonder what will happen when my CP increases even more.

A: Sleep is a complicated topic. In fact, it is easier to analyze, treat and predict the dynamic of cancer, diabetes or emphysema where nearly all effects are linear and simpler. The best way to predict the effects of higher CP is to experience it.

As about dreams, I believe that there are dozens of other factors that are more important for health and wellbeing of a person than remembering dreams. Yes, most people, when they get up to 30-60 s for their morning CPs, do not remember dreams (usually nothing at all). These people usually start with about 15-20 s CP. However, at lower CPs, you can have the opposite effect. With about 10 s CP, you may not have certain chemical reactions that promote your ability to recall dreams. With about 15-20 s, these reactions reappear and you are able to remember dreams. However, at higher CPs, you do not remember dreams for some other causes.

You can achieve better dream recall by taking large doses of vitamin B6 (pyridoxine). This effect will probably be present at any CP level.

Q: I am under the firm belief that polyphasic sleeping is the best way for health. What this means is sleeping in many short periods per 24 hours instead of sleeping for one long period. I used to sleep 12 hours a night and be all groggy when I woke up. If I sleep in a 4 then 2 hour period or two 3 hour periods or better yet three 1 hour periods, I feel much more vital and healthy than before. Also my dreams are more healing, and more dream recall because of the connection to the waking consciousness. My waking life is more happy because of the connection to the dream consciousness and my "soul". Pretty much I think that long periods of being awake stress the nervous system and cause the widespread unnatural 7-10 hour sleep periods we see. I believe that one should sleep no more than 6 hours in a row. The ideal sleep for a working 8 hour day man would be a 4 hour core sleep and a 2 hour "nap". and a man with a flexible schedule should sleep in as much a polyphasic manner as he dares. I don't know how much polyphasic is too much, but it seems to increase restfulness and alertness with less total sleep (e.g., the Uberman cycle is only 2 hours total), increase the time in the day to do things, and increase one's health, so it's all good.

A: There is some anthropological evidence that suggests that it has been common for humans to have "fluid" sleep patterns that is similar to polyphasic sleep. I do not currently have enough data to suggest polyphasic sleep to all people. Maybe it can be a good option for most or only some people.

Q: I have a query on my sleep. Basically when I do not have to get up for work, I am sleeping 9 hours, but the last 1.5 hours are broken and light. I cannot seem to get out of bed. I try to, but I cannot. I just go back to bed and have broken and light sleep. This makes me feel pretty miserable in the mornings., and I think I generally feel slow, drained, and tired, for most of the day. Do you have any advice for me? My MCP is around 35, sometimes 40, not straining, just when my diaphragm starts to really move. What do you think? I sleep on an incline; mouth tape; take vitamin D, fish oil, zinc, and magnesium; and exercise not as much as I can, just when I feel like it. I eat healthy, the Paleo diet mainly.

A: You probably did not measure your CP correctly. With morning CP 35 s, you should have around 6 hours of sleep. Also, it is nearly impossible to get MCP 30+ with nearly no exercise. Your real MCP is about 15-20 seconds. It is common for people who learn the Buteyko method to measure their CPs incorrectly and claim twice larger numbers.

Concerning your optimum action plan, it is too hard to tell due to insufficient information you provided. Apart from more exercise, you may have problems with low or marginally low iodine or a lack of deep stages of sleep or too low blood glucose levels in the morning. Earthing can solve the problem if your body positive charge is a problem.

Q: This might be a stupid question. What does sleep do for you? Why do people need sleep? I heard that brains are more active when people are asleep, so why can't people just rest instead of sleeping?

A: That is a hard question. There are many changes during sleep that are not possible to achieve in active mental states. The brain is not just less active during sleep, but there are brain areas and wave patterns that appear or become more active or predominant, while others disappear or get reduced. Sleep does many things, and mammals lose appetite and die without sleep in 1-2 weeks.

Q: I just want to ask about the mechanics of sleep with high CP levels. For instance, sleep occurs with various cycles happening, deep sleep, REM phase, etc. If one's CP is higher, then does this reduce the time taken for each cycle to complete?

A: With a higher CP, sleep gets shorter usually due to an elimination of one whole cycle. Duration of sleep stages, as well as the presence of REM sleep, remain the same. As a result, most people, when their morning CP gets higher, notice a step-like reduction. For example, with 20 s morning CP, one's sleep was 7 hours. When the same person achieved over 30 s for the morning CP, his or her sleep was reduced by 1 hour due to elimination of the whole cycle of sleep.

Note that some people can have disturbed sleep due to sleep apnea or other causes. In such cases, the total number and duration of deep stages of sleep can be reduced causing daytime sleepiness and fatigue.

Q: Is it OK to go to sleep at a routine time if I'm always tired and ready to sleep at that time?

A: It is good for sleep hygiene to get sleepy at the same time and to have a routine. However, with increasing CPs, sleep naturally shortens. One can stay awake longer and can naturally wake up earlier too (without a desire to sleep more).

Q: Is it healthy to be able to sleep so deeply that even a severely heavy thunderstorm can't wake one up (in same position for 5 hrs for instance)?

A: It is healthy to have deep stages of sleep and the REM sleep afterwards. It is unhealthy not to have them.

It is unhealthy to sleep more than 4 hours in the same position since prolonged immobility makes breathing heavier and reduces one's CP.

Q: I find this so amazing. Have you had experience with people able to sleep only 2-3 hours per day besides Dr. Buteyko himself? It must be really strange to be able to go on at night while everybody else is sleeping and probably takes a lot of getting used to?

A: I have had many students (some of them in their 60's and 70's) who got over 50 s for their morning CPs. All of them were happy with about 4 hours of natural sleep. I had nights with 2 hours of sleep without any desire to sleep more, and months with 4 hours of sleep per night. To get there is the same as to breaking through the morning 40 s CP threshold. This is the hardest goal in breathing retraining, especially if you do not know how to do it (there are some techniques that help).

Q: How fast can one adapt to 2 hours of sleep a night on average using breathing techniques?

A: 2 hours of sleep comes naturally with about 2-3 min CP, so there is no need to adapt to that. Just get over 2 min CP and enjoy your short sleep naturally.

Q: Which breathing techniques do you consider as the best for the goal of significantly reducing sleep duration, and which way of learning do you recommend?

A: With less than 20-25 s for the current CP (over 90% of all modern people), it is easier to start with breathing devices (the Frolov device or an Amazing DIY breathing device). Once you have over 25 s CP, in addition, you can learn the Buteyko breathing exercises. For example, you can use the book "Advanced Buteyko Breathing Exercises".

7.2 Swaddling during sleep

Q: When I use swaddling, I wake up at about 3 am and cannot sleep. What is wrong? What can I do?

A: If you use swaddling, but wake up at night (e.g., at 3-4 am) and cannot sleep, this can be a sign that you started to hyperventilate and your vest or belts were trying to prevent overbreathing. In this case, you need to analyze all those positive and negative factors that we considered above.

If you still experience this problem, you need to use something similar to the wake-up method described above. In other words, when you wake up at 3 am, practice a breathing session, increase your CP and make breathing lighter. Then you can go to sleep while being swaddled again.

You may also reduce the intensity of swaddling (making it less tight) and see if it is easier to tolerate, but still effective enough for your morning CP.

Q: If we wore a weighted vest, would we get the same high quality sleep on our backs with these vests on as we would by sleeping on our stomachs? If we wore these vests sitting up, couldn't we doubly suppress our breathing and get even better sleep?

A: Each factor works independently by itself. Belts or swaddling will help to reduce breathing for any position. Sleep positions have their own contribution. We get the best morning CPs while sleeping sitting, with slightly lower CP numbers for prone and the left positions. The CP drop will be small, if any, for the supine position if swaddling is tight enough.

The same is probably true for extra weight. You can get benefits from anything heavy that is on your chest, while you sleep in a supine position. Likely, you can get even more benefits from the same weight when you sleep on your stomach.

Q: I found that if I use one main belt, I become an abdominal breather. However, if I apply a second belt below the main one, I get upper chest breathing. What should I do?

A: You are on the border so that your breathing, after the main belt, can go in both directions: it can become abdominal, but if you add a belt to restrict abdominal breathing, you become an upper chest breather. In this case, I suggest you try only one belt for 4-5 nights in row in order to acquire (or adapt to) abdominal breathing. Later, especially when you get higher morning CPs, apply an additional belt below the main one, with mild pressure only, and monitor the effects. If you start with a light abdominal pressure only, you will still have abdominal breathing during sleep. Then you can gradually increase pressure, and use more and tighter belts, while preserving abdominal or diaphragmatic breathing.

Alternatively, you can make a swaddling vest that solves this problem since it provides a good restriction for the middle chest and prevents expansion of the rib cage during inhalations.

7.3 Overbreathing during sleep

Q: I start to hyperventilate after 1 hour of sleep. What should I do?

A: As we discussed above, this is common in severely sick people due to multiple health problems that make breathing heavier. You need to get up to 20 s CP as soon as possible using all available methods and techniques. Then you will not have this problem with overbreathing after 1 hour of sleep.

In the meantime, you can try to sleep sitting, and/or do breathing sessions during sleep, and/or use swaddling.

Q: Since I've started doing Buteyko every night, I've woken up in the middle of sleep with a stuffed nose and dyspnea. I'm not sleeping on my back anymore, and I also meditate and exercise. What's wrong? Or is this normal?

A: It is unclear if your past sleep was better or worse, and by how much. If your sleep is worse now, it is not normal. If you practice a lot of reduced breathing (e.g., over 2 hours per day) and wake up at 3-4 am, this can take place due to the onset of overbreathing. Hyperventilation during sleep speedily wakes up diligent breathing students. You need to add more physical exercise and solve other problems related to your low morning CP. Once your morning CP is higher, you should be able to sleep throughout the whole night without interruptions. If your morning CP gets up to 20-25 s, then both symptoms, a stuffy nose and dyspnea, should disappear.

Q: How can I avoid mouth breathing at night if I have nasal polyps? Lying down blocks my nose completely. Can I still get a higher CP and avoid surgery?

A: In nearly all cases of nasal polyps, the surgery can be avoided. You need 30 s morning CP (20+ s for the morning CP is the first goal). Breathwork with the breathing device (either the Frolov breathing device or DIY device) is the optimum way to start. If the nose gets blocked after transition to the horizontal position, try to sleep sitting. With higher CPs, your problem will become reduced as well as the time of its onset. These are general or long-term goals.

In the meantime, try to sleep in sitting position, and/or use swaddling and other methods that increase your morning CP.

Q: 1. What is the closest to bed time that one should perform high intensity exercise?
2. ...And working on the computer?

A: 1. The effects of high intensity physical exercise on sleep are very individual. These effects usually depend on how physical exercise influences the sympathetic nervous system. Some people are ok to have intensive exercise, even games, 20-30 min before sleep, while others may remain overexcited even after 4-5 hours. If someone did not play active sport games for weeks or months, he or she may remain overexcited for the main part of the day, for up to 12 hours. This means that intensive or stimulating exercise at noon time may affect sleep over 12 hours later. Thus, adaptation and individual differences are large factors here.

2. Computers are generally less influential, but it depends a lot on the nature of your computer work and degree of addiction if you play computer games. For many people, computer games can have a strong negative effect of the nervous system, breathing and brain waves during sleep.

7.5 Sleep conditions

Q: If a bed is too soft to provide good sleep hygiene, would it be a good idea to sleep on the floor (covered by 2 layers of thin blanket) instead (provided the floor is sufficiently cleaned)? Or would that be problematic for whatever reasons (if, for example, as I suspect, too many airborne particles might accumulate on the ground despite all cleaning)?

A: Yes. You can sleep on the floor with 1-2 thin blankets. Air quality is about the same: on the bed or on the floor. Sleeping sitting is even a better option.

Q: Do you think that sleeping on a slightly inclined platform, with the head end raised approx 10-20 degrees, would have a beneficial effect on sleeping?

A: Yes, *inclined sleep therapy* helps to reduce many symptoms, especially for those people who have poor sleep quality. I mean those people who spend more than 10 min trying to fall asleep and/or wake up at night for more than 10 minutes.

Q: I saw that a good sleeping position is lying on your left. I've been sleeping on my right side because I was told that things (foods) drain in that direction. I also heard that sleeping on your right would give more space for the heart (sleeping on left side would press the heart more). I learned this through Chinese and Ayurvedic Medicine as well as Macrobiotic theory. I would like to see if you have any comment about this. Thank you very much.

A: There are many theories and justifications for different sleep positions. My ideas and suggestions are based on clinical experience of Soviet and Russian Buteyko doctors with over 200,000 patients. We care about breathing and O2 levels in the body cells using these parameters as the main criteria for choosing best sleep positions.

Q: I was thinking that sleeping in a vibrating/massaging chair could be very healthy. Any experience with this?

A: Yes, there is some limited positive experience. Application of shaking or vibration devices helps to improve metabolism and reduce effects of immobility during sleep. One can attach to a bed, with straps or other methods, even a simple fan. Many people know and notice that their digestion and GI signs are improved when they have long bus or train trips due to hours of body vibrations. Dr. Buteyko mentioned positive effects of shaking/vibrations on breathing and health.

Q: It might be a silly question, but still, why do we need fresh air while sleeping or doing breathing exercises. Doesn't it mean that fresh air brings more O2 and lowers CO2. On the contrary, there are less O2 and more CO2 in a stuffy room that eventually should lead human body to better oxygenation. So, in order to adapt our brain and whole body to higher CO2 level, looks like we need to spend more time in stuffy environment?

A: The stalest rooms around us have negligible changes in O2 and CO2 to cause any noticeable physiological effects. One needs the Training Mask, the Frolov device, the DIY device, or sleeping under the blanket with a tiny hole (or a high altitude tent), in order to get a 1-2% CO2 increase and about the same O2 drop in the lungs.

Q: Would it increase O2 and improve sleep if you sleep with a gas mask on and still taped mouth? So nasal breathing but with resistance from the mask?

A: Yes, this can help to increase morning CP. There are published studies with positive effects of additional dead space to improve sleeping patterns in people with sleep apnea.

Q: Is the need for time spent outdoors at all relevant to sunlight, meaning that time spent outdoors in the sun would be more productive than time outdoors after dark?

A: Maybe there are effects of sunlight on calcium metabolism and this helps some people to sleep better. However, most people are unlikely to notice any good effects of sun on their sleep. Beyond a certain limit (about 20-30 minutes), radiation due to direct sun rays usually causes cellular damage and CP drop.

Q: Why sleeping outdoors is better?

A: It is hard to tell why outdoors makes sleep better: Earth's magnetic field, or more natural environment, or ions, or grounding, or a combination of such factors.

7.6 Sleep positions

Q: I tape my mouth at night but do nothing to prevent sleeping on the back besides laying on my side until I fall asleep. If I do an hour of exercise that day then shouldn't my body adapt to that CP the next day anyway? How important is to prevent sleeping on the back? Some days I feel okay the next day and some days I feel awful no matter how much exercise and breath work I do.

A: The effects of supine sleep are individual.

If overbreathing is accompanied by increased sensitivity to allergic triggers, then overbreathing combined with poor quality of air, amplifies the negative effects of dust, dust mites, mold, and so on. For this person, supine sleep will trigger an allergic reaction during sleep.

Somebody with a sinus infection can first experience a slight CP drop (e.g., from 20 to 17) due to a supine sleep. This slight overbreathing makes the immune system weak causing a quick advance of pathogens in sinuses. The nose gets blocked, he or she starts mouth breathing. This will further reduce his or her CP to about 10 s CP in the morning, with headaches and a blocked nose.

For an asthmatic, supine sleep can increase ventilation to the levels causing more inflammation in the airways, wheezing, extra mucus production, coughing, and other symptoms.

Therefore, if supine sleep triggers some other processes, its effects are very large with up to 2-4 times decrease in their CPs. In other words, they start to breathe about 2-4 times more air.

For relatively healthy people (or those who do not suffer from some additional or triggered events and symptoms), the effects of supine sleep are less strong. However, supine sleep can still take from you up to 30-50% of your evening CP.

Q: I have always slept on my side. But now that I have been trying to learn Buteyko breathing I have become more interested in my breathing habits during sleep (I do tape my mouth for sleeping. I have been doing this for about 3 weeks now).

What I have discovered is that if I feel any "air distress" at all, it is immediately relieved by turning onto my back. It's very clear for me that this is true (again, this is with mouth taped). It seems that my urge to breathe, my breathing rate, the depth of my breath--these all are reduced if I roll over on to my back.

So my question is: What exactly is wrong with sleeping on the back? If it is because people tend to open their mouths, then I understand and agree--mouth breathing must be avoided. But do you still claim that sleeping on the back is bad even when breathing through the nose?

A: Of course, it is easier to breathe more while sleeping on the back. This is the reason why supine sleep is so addictive. It makes breathing deeper regardless of the route: mouth or nose. For other positions, when you sleep and breathe, you need to lift a main part of your trunk with each inhalation. For supine sleep you do not do that (or you lift much less weight). Hence, supine sleep encourages deeper breathing and larger ventilation even with nose breathing, and mouth breathing is just an additional after-effect of sleeping on one's back.

Q: What if one elevates the upper half of his body (maybe using pillows) to 30-45 degrees (instead of 90 degrees which is the sitting position)? Will that be beneficial? Can he sleep on his back and still have good results this way or does he still need to sleep on the side?

A: The reclining position is almost the same as supine sleep and causes low body O2, unless one uses belts to prevent chest breathing (and maybe another belt below).

Q: Even if someone elevates the upper half of his body 75 degrees (instead of 90 which is the sitting position) this is still considered as supine and therefore bad?

A: Over 80 degrees would be ok.

Q: If I sleep in a sitting position all the time, my CP should not drop at all due to sleeping hyperventilation right. Is this correct?

A: Yes, your CP should not drop much or at all.

Q: I have a doubt about the sleeping postures. For many years I have been practicing lucid dreaming, and for that it is usually recommended to sleep on the right side. It seems that sleeping on the right side allows for a more lucid consciousness while dreaming: "people had three times as many lucid dreams when sleeping on their right sides (as the lion doth?) than when sleeping on their left sides." lucidity.com How can I reconcile with the recommendations given here? Is it really that bad from the breathing perspective the right side sleep?

A: For over 97% of people, sleeping on the right side is not as bad as supine sleep, but it still reduces body oxygenation. Healthy people (here we measure health by body O2 content) do not remember any dreams, and I do not think that lucid dreaming or even watching full color movies all night provides any criteria or guarantee of good physical or mental health. I think that solving problems with chronic diseases and an ability to perform much better in physical, mental, and spiritual areas in real life are more important than dreams during sleep.

Q: I kind of have an odd way of viewing this. They say here that body oxygen in the Supine position is 50%. Wouldn't this be a good thing meaning you are actually resting your body and not having to use as much O2. Hence you. it seems like that by sleeping in the other positions you are getting more oxygen, but who knows you could just be "using" more oxygen. I am just here thinking outside the box. If any doctors or scientists out there could look into these things that would be awesome. meaning "how much oxygen do we really need while sleeping"? "If running at 50% oxygen helps conserve energy and repair things that you can't see on the graph", how did these subjects do the next day being the Supine Versus Prone. Are they equally aware/awake, in all sorts, brain activity/physical activity/memory?

A: You may think that you are "outside the box", but evolution and Nature created the human body to function in conditions of high CO2. Therefore, when we go outside the box, we suffer from heart attacks, seizures, asthma attacks, growth of cancer tumors and much more. For research, you need to look at the measurable sleep effects (or effects of heavy breathing during sleep) on sick and severely sick people: http://www.normalbreathing.com/index-MorningHV.php. I do not see anything "helpful" in this Sleep Heavy Breathing Effect. It does not train the human body.

Yes, training at high altitude, or using the Training Mask or breathing devices, all create mild hypoxia as well. But these types of training are accompanied by higher CO2, whereas supine sleep causes both deficiencies - low O2 and low CO2 at the same time. That creates health misery with later effects on everything including brain activity/physical activity/memory. You can confirm these ideas yourself by testing different positions, and possibly even measuring the CP.

Q: Why CP drops while sleeping, especially in supine position?

A: Dr. Buteyko suggested that breathing during supine sleep is unrestricted. The chest and belly movements have less resistance in comparison with other horizontal positions. That causes overbreathing and lower CPs.

Q: For a number of months now, I have been sleeping with the head of my bed raised six inches. As a result, I sleep more soundly and wake up more refreshed. According to the work of Andrew K. Fletcher on "Inclined Bed Therapy," an inclined bed improves circulation throughout the body even in the lower legs. The science behind it is intriguing. I'd like to see a study of body oxygenation done with people sleeping in the inclined position. I'd hypothesize that oxygenation might approach 90%.

A: Inclined beds help those students whose CPs drop at night due to sleeping problems (inability to fall asleep within 10 min or waking up for more than 10 min at night). It is definitely a simple and important technique to improve ones health and reduce effects of insomnia. It may be effective for other people as well.

Q: What do you think about the "V-shape bed" also called the Pilates bed invented by J.H.Pilates in 1934 and claimed to provide the fullest and most complete relaxation of all muscles, shown on http://geoffjones.com/pilates-bed/

A: This bed changes all 4 classical positions making it impossible to have a pure supine or pure prone posture. Instead, it creates 2 supine and 2 prone sleep positions. Both supine positions for this bed (with inclines to the left and to the right) will make breathing heavy and the CP low. But sleeping on the chest (with a right or left incline) for this bed should work equally well for easier breathing and higher CP.

Q: I find I can't do reduced breathing when lying in bed at night. It's as if my breathing is as reduced as it can be. I can do it sitting up to a mild degree. How can I stop the breath difficulties in the night?

A: Reduced breathing in a horizontal position is possible and works if you do it on the left side or chest, and you do it when you are sleepy (or deprived of sleep). Then the body has a positive reaction to the transition into a horizontal position. There are possible chemicals, such as hormones, that favor your transition into a horizontal position. However, if you do not feel sleepy, it could be impossible to reduce your breathing since the body "rebels" against this body posture.

7.7 Sleep and breathing in world class athletes

Q: According to researchers Martin Miller and Judd Biasiotto, world class athletes sleep an average of 520 minutes per night - 8.75 hours a night. That is approximately an hour more sleep than what researchers Frederick Backeland and Ernest Hartmann found for the average person. According to those researchers, the average person sleeps 7.5 hours per night. Does that mean world class athletes have an MCP around 20 s? I would guess that world class athletes should have an MCP of at least 60 s. Otherwise, I would guess that all gold medals at the Olympics could easily be won by Buteyko athletes.

A: World class athletes also have high rates of asthma, cancer, diabetes, heart disease, and other health problems. They are nearly as sick as the ordinary population because their usual body oxygenation is around 20-25 s (slightly better than average numbers). Therefore, they are only marginally healthier.

As about effects of breathing retraining, better or easier breathing improves sport performance mainly for endurance events such as long distance running - see the Tarahumara-runners section on this page: www.normalbreathing.com/s/breathing-techniques-for-running.php.

Most importantly, high body O2 levels, due to easier breathing 24/7, increases one's ability to train harder without injuries What I mean here is the following. In my early years, I spent over 10 years training, living, and traveling with numerous world and sometimes Olympic champions from national and other top teams. The adaptation of the human body to nearly maximum possible intensity and duration of training is a CP-dependent process.

At lower CPs (e.g., less than 30 s), this process is called "wear": the training effect is accompanied by destructive processes in muscles and body organs due to chronic tissue hypoxia (low body oxygenation) with chronic stress for the immune system and other systems of the body.

At higher CPs (over 30 s, or better yet, over 50 s), the body also adapts to exercise but without these injurious effects that cause wear on the organs and tissues. This is the reason why after completing their sport career, most professional athletes feel sick and become plagued by chronic health problems with further reduction in their CPs due to less exercise that played some positive role in the past.

Recommended reading

The Secret World of Sleep: The Surprising Science of the Mind at Rest (MacSci), by Penelope A. Lewis (Kindle and hardcover) - http://www.amazon.com/The-Secret-World-Sleep-ebook/dp/B00E2PZTG4/

The Effortless Sleep Method:The Incredible New Cure for Insomnia and Chronic Sleep Problems, by Sasha Stephens (Kindle and paperback) - http://www.amazon.com/The-Effortless-Sleep-Method-ebook/dp/B004UC4ZNM/

To increase your body oxygenation, learn and/or refine your Buteyko breathing exercises using this 2013 Amazon book (Kindle and paperback): "Advanced Buteyko Breathing Exercises" - http://www.amazon.com/Advanced-Buteyko-Breathing-Exercises-ebook/dp/B00CAXAKAA/. It considers, in detail, many unique topics and effects that are not present in any other book.

Do you know that, in relation to foods and diets, it is more important what eats you rather than a modern obsession with "you are what you eat"? There are clear and specific numerous signs of ideal or normal digestion, which include a clean tongue (no white or yellow coating to scrape) and no need to use toilet paper (no soiling). If soiling is present, that means that one has poor GI flora, and this reduces body oxygenation and reduces your CP during sleep. The PDF book "Perfect Digestion" deals with these symptoms and explains how to achieve no soiling and other signs of great GI health. You can get this book from NormalBreathing site: How to Improve Digestion with Lifestyle and Higher Body O2 - http://www.normalbreathing.com/how-to/how-to-improve-digestion.php or go on Smashwords where you can find many other formats (such as EPUB, Kindle, LRF, PDB, etc.) "Perfect Digestion" - https://www.smashwords.com/books/view/327725

Please, feel free to leave you honest review on the Amazon page of this book.

Other books by Dr. Artour Rakhimov

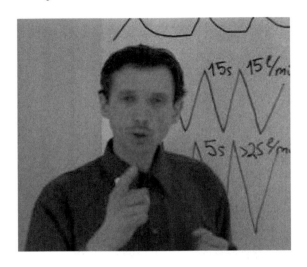

- "Advanced Buteyko Breathing Exercises" 2013 - PDF and Amazon book
- "Cystic Fibrosis Life Expectancy: 30, 50, 70, ..." 2012 - Amazon book
- "Doctors Who Cure Cancer" 2012 - Amazon book
- "Yoga Benefits Are in Breathing Less" 2012 - Amazon book
- "Crohn's Disease and Colitis: Hidden Triggers and Symptoms" 2012 - Amazon book
- "Perfect Digestion" 2013 - PDF book
- "How to Use Frolov Breathing Device (Instructions)" 2012 - PDF and Amazon book (120 pages)
- "Amazing DIY Breathing Device" 2010-2012 - PDF and Amazon book
- "Doctor Buteyko Lecture at the Moscow State University" 2009 (55 pages; Translation from Russian with Dr. A. Rakhimov's comments)
- "Normal Breathing: the Key to Vital Health" 2009 (The most comprehensive book on the Buteyko breathing retraining method; over 190,000 words; 305 pages)

Printed in Great Britain
by Amazon